Pathology of the Human Em
and Previable Fetus

D.K. Kalousek N. Fitch B.A. Paradice

Pathology of the Human Embryo and Previable Fetus

An Atlas

With 258 Illustrations in 361 Parts Including 17 Color Plates

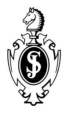

Springer-Verlag
New York Berlin Heidelberg
London Paris Tokyo Hong Kong

Dagmar K. Kalousek, MD, FRCPC, FCCMG
Professor, Department of Pathology, The University of British Columbia and BC
Children's Hospital, Vancouver, V6H 3V4, Canada

Naomi Fitch, MD, PhD
Visiting Assistant Professor, Department of Pathology, The University of British
Columbia, Lady Davis Institute, Sir Mortimer B. Davis Jewish General Hospital,
Montreal, H3T 1E2, Canada

Barbara A. Paradice, ART
Laboratory Technologist, Embryopathology Unit, BC Children's Hospital, Vancouver,
V6H 3V4, Canada

Library of Congress Cataloging-in-Publication Data
Kalousek, Dagmar K.
   Pathology of the human embryo and previable fetus : an atlas /
Dagmar K. Kalousek, Naomi Fitch, Barbara Paradice.
      p. cm.
   ISBN 0-387-97168-8
   1. Fetus—Abnormalities. 2. Human embryo—Abnormalities.
3. Fetus—Examination. 4. Placenta—Examination. I. Fitch, Naomi.
II. Paradice, Barbara. III. Title.
   [DNLM: 1. Fetus—pathology—atlases. 2. Placenta—pathology—
atlases. 3. Pregnancy Complications—pathology—atlases. WQ 17
K142R]
RG626.K35   1990
618.3′2071—dc20
DNLM/DLC
for Library of Congress   89-21935

Typeset by Publishers Service, Bozeman, Montana.
Printed and bound by Arcata Graphics/Halliday, West Hanover, Massachusetts.
Printed in the United States of America.

9 8 7 6 5 4 3 2 1

ISBN 0-387-97168-8 Springer-Verlag New York Berlin Heidelberg
ISBN 3-540-97168-8 Springer-Verlag Berlin Heidelberg New York

D.K. Kalousek   To my teachers and my family—my mother, Jan, Joseph, Andrea, and Ingrid

N. Fitch   To two wonderful biologists and teachers, Dr. N.J. Berrill and Dr. F.C. Fraser, and to my children, Tamara and Anna

B.A. Paradice   To Dr. Betty J. Poland who introduced me to Embryofetopathology and to my husband, Allen

Preface

This book is designed primarily for anatomic pathologists to facilitate their task of accurately diagnosing embryos and fetuses. A detailed examination of the products of spontaneous and induced abortions is necessary for accurate genetic counseling and for establishing the risk for specific abnormalities or another spontaneous pregnancy loss in the future.

The growing interest in the defects of early development reflects the profound change in general life-style. In the past, spontaneous abortions were considered a common, usually sporadic event in a patient's reproductive history. Only reassurance and encouragement were given to the patient and scant attention was paid to the detailed pathology of the abortus. Nowadays, however, as a result of reliable methods of contraception and of the availability of reliable prenatal diagnosis for chromosome abnormalities more frequent in advanced maternal age, significant numbers of parents plan to have pregnancies later in their reproductive life. Consequently, in a case of spontaneous abortion, the question of "cause" and of "future risk" of recurrence of abortion or an abnormal infant is particularly important. In the era of more elaborate and accurate prenatal diagnostic tests, the pathologist examining products of conception has a primary responsibility to detect, in both spontaneous and induced abortions, any developmental abnormality that would indicate an increased risk of multifactorial, chromosomal, and single gene disorders in a subsequent child. Following pregnancy termination after a first or a second trimester prenatal diagnosis of a defective conceptus, the pathologist is not only responsible for confirming the abnormal development of the conceptus but also for correlating the morphologic findings with ultrasound, cytogenetic, biochemical, and DNA diagnosis and making a correct final diagnosis to facilitate appropriate prenatal care in the next pregnancy.

Clinicians—medical geneticists, obstetricians, and sonologists—will find this text useful for its visualization of specific morphologic lesions and illustrations of the variable expression of genetic syndromes in embryonic and fetal periods.

The book is divided into three major parts. The first part provides a general review of normal embryonic and fetal development. The second deals with abortion and the basic approach to the examination of aborted embryos and fetuses. In the third part, pathologic findings detected on examination of products of conception are discussed. Practical issues of specimen collection and examination are summarized in the Appendices. It is important to note that, in this book's illustrations, the developmental, not the gestational age (see Chapter 3), of embryos and fetuses is given.

Dagmar K. Kalousek
Naomi Fitch
Barbara A. Paradice

Acknowledgments

We are very grateful to Dr. Clarke Fraser, Dr. Wes Tyson, Dr. Jan Friedman, and Dr. Enid Gilbert-Barness for their many helpful suggestions. We are indebted to Miss Vicky Earle, medical artist, for her fine drawings and Miss Miranda Tsai for her help with manuscript preparation. We would also like to thank the members of the Department of Pathology for their unfailing cooperation and support. The authors would also like to acknowledge the generous support and help of the book production staff of Springer-Verlag.

Contents

C. Pathology of Embryonic, Fetal, and Placental Development

A. Normal Embryonic and Fetal Development

bleeding during pregnancy or at delivery. Cervical pregnancy, in which implantation occurs in the cervical canal, is very rare. It is likely, however, that some of these pregnancies are not recognized because the conceptus is expelled early in gestation. Implantation occurring outside the uterus results in an *ectopic pregnancy*. The majority of ectopic implantations occur in the Fallopian tube. Ectopic tubal pregnancies frequently result in rupture of the Fallopian tube and hemorrhage followed by the death of the conceptus. Ectopic pregnancies occurring on the surface of the ovary, on the peritoneum of the broad ligament, on the mesentery of the intestine, or in the rectouterine pouch are much rarer.

Many conceptuses are unable to implant due to their abnormal genetic make-up and are therefore lost during the first week of development (Chapter III).

The Second Week of Development (Stage 5)

Implantation of the blastocyst continues during the second week while significant morphological changes occur in the inner cell mass. The second week of development is sometimes called *the period of twos* (Crowley, 1974) because a *bilaminar embryonic disc* forms, *amniotic* and *primary yolk sac cavities* develop, and *two layers of trophoblast—cytotrophoblast* and *syncytiotrophoblast*—differentiate (Fig. I-1b).

The two-layered disc arrangement of the embryo that separates the blastocyst cavity into two unequal parts—the smaller amniotic cavity and the larger primary yolk cavity (Stage 5)—becomes evident during the early part of the second week. The thick layer of embryonic cells bordering the amniotic cavity is called the *epiblast* (ectoderm) and the thin layer bordering the primary yolk cavity is called the *hypoblast* (endoderm).

Rapid proliferation of the trophoblast and its differentiation into two layers, an inner *cytotrophoblast* and an outer *syncytiotrophoblast*, is an important feature of this period. Although the trophoblast continues to penetrate deeper into the endometrium, the differentiating inner cell mass is never deeper than a few millimeters from the surface of the endometrium. At the end of the second week, the implantation site may be recognized as a small elevated area of endometrium with a central pore occupied by a blood clot.

The Third Week of Development (Stages 6–9)

The third week is characterized by the formation of the primitive streak (Stage 6) and three germ layers (ectoderm, mesoderm, and endoderm), from which all tissues and organs of the embryo develop.

At first the *primitive streak* (Fig. I-2) appears as an opaque node caused by the proliferation of ectodermal cells at the caudal end of the embryonal disc. The cells of the primitive streak undergo extensive multiplication and expand laterally, caudally, and in cephalic direction between the ectoderm and endoderm of the embryonic disc to form the *embryonic mesoblast*, the progenitor of mesoderm.

While the primitive streak is giving rise to the embryonic mesoblast, a solid cord of cells grows cephalically from the *primitive knot*, which is the cephalic end of the primitive streak, and becomes attached to the endoderm below the point of fused ectoderm and endoderm in the region of the future buccopharyngeal membrane. This cord of cells is known as the *notochord* (Fig. I-2). The notochord is the base around which the vertebral column and the base of the skull develop, and it also defines the craniocaudal axis of embryonic development (Stage 7).

A thickening of the ectodermal cells lying above the developing notochord gives rise to the *neural plate*. The neural plate is the first part of the nervous system to appear. The neural plate becomes depressed along the long axis of the embryo to form the *neural groove* which is flanked by *neural folds* (Stage 8) (Fig. I-3a). As the neural groove deepens, the neural folds elevate and fuse in the midline to form the *neural tube* (Fig. I-3b). The process of fusion begins in the region of the future embryonic neck and extends towards the cephalic and caudal ends of the embryo. Fusion is completed during the fourth week of development. The neural tube ultimately will give rise to the central nervous system. The cephalic end will dilate to form the forebrain, midbrain, and hindbrain. The remainder of the neural tube will become the spinal cord.

While the neural tube is developing, the mesoderm present on either side of the midline of the embryo, the *paraxial mesoderm*, undergoes segmentation, by which it becomes

---

Fig. I-1. Diagram showing formation of the zygote (a) and bilaminar embryonic disc (b) in the second week of development.

Fig. I-2. Diagram showing the development of the primitive streak and the notochord.

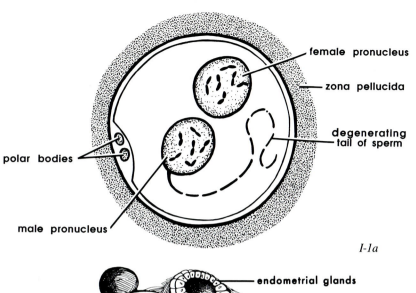

female pronucleus

zona pellucida

degenerating tail of sperm

polar bodies

male pronucleus

I-1a

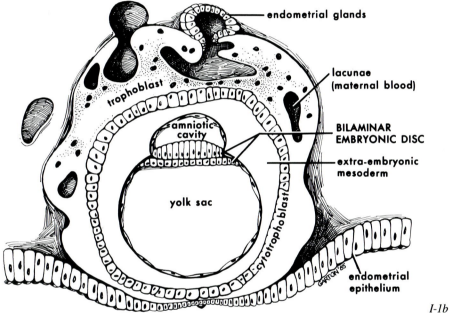

endometrial glands

lacunae (maternal blood)

trophoblast

amniotic cavity

BILAMINAR EMBRYONIC DISC

extra-embryonic mesoderm

yolk sac

cytotrophoblast

endometrial epithelium

I-1b

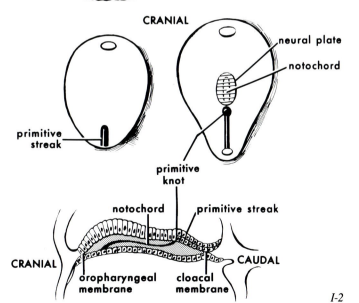

CRANIAL

neural plate

notochord

primitive streak

primitive knot

notochord

primitive streak

CRANIAL

CAUDAL

oropharyngeal membrane

cloacal membrane

I-2

divided into segmental blocks or *somites*. This process starts during Stage 9. Eventually, there are approximately 43 pairs of somites. Each somite later differentiates into the bones, cartilage, and ligaments of the vertebral column as well as into skeletal voluntary muscles and the dermis and subcutaneous tissue of the skin. The *intermediate mesoderm*, the mesodermal tissue present on both sides of the embryo between the paraxial mesoderm and the lateral mesoderm, gives rise to portions of the urogenital system. The *lateral mesoderm* is involved in the development of the pericardial, pleural, and peritoneal cavities, as well as the muscle of the diaphragm.

The embryonic mesoblast (see above) also gives rise to a *primitive cardiovascular system* during the third week of development. Blood vessel formation begins in the extraembryonic mesoderm of the yolk sac, the connecting stalk, and the chorion. It is followed by the development of vessels in the embryo two days later. The primitive heart forms from mesenchymal cells that differentiate into muscular and connective tissue in the cardiogenic area. The connection of the primitive heart tube with blood vessels takes place towards the end of the third week, after which the embryo's blood begins to circulate.

As the embryo progressively changes shape from a disc to a tube exhibiting cranial and caudal ends with a head and a tail, *endoderm*, the third germ layer, becomes incorporated into the interior of the embryo, where it contributes to the epithelial components of most internal organs.

Further development of the placenta, specifically formation of chorionic villi, takes place in the third week. *Primary chorionic villi* acquire cores of mesenchyme and become *secondary chorionic villi*. Before the end of the third week, capillaries develop in the villi, transforming them into *tertiary chorionic villi*. At the same time, the cytotrophoblast cells of the chorionic villi penetrate the layer of syncytiotrophoblast to form a *cytotrophoblastic shell*, which attaches the chorionic sac to the endometrial tissues (Hamilton et al., 1978).

The Fourth Week of Development (Stages 10–12)

During the fourth week of development, the embryo, which measures 2 to 5 mm, is recognizable by the naked eye. At stage 10, the embryo (22–24 days) is almost straight and the existing 4 to 12 somites produce conspicuous surface elevations (Fig. I-3b). The neural tube is closed in the area adjacent to the somites but is widely open at the rostral and caudal neuropores. The first and second pair of branchial arches become visible.

During Stage 11, a slight curve is produced in the embryo by a folding of the head and tail. The heart is seen as a large ventral prominence. The rostral neuropore continues to close, and branchial arches 1 and 2 are evident (Fig. I-4). In addition, the optic vesicles and otic pits are developing, and the mesonephric ducts and nephric tubules appear.

Stage 12 is characterized by three pairs of branchial arches, complete closure of the rostral hemisphere, and the presence of recognizable upper limb buds on the ventrolateral body wall. The otic pits, the primordia of the inner ears, are also clearly visible (Fig. I-5). The growth of the forebrain produces a prominent elevation of the head, and further folding of the embryo in the longitudinal plane gives the embryo a characteristic C-shaped curvature. Narrowing of the connection between the embryo and the yolk sac produces a body stalk containing one umbilical vein and two umbilical arteries.

Fig. I-3. (a) Diagram of the trilaminar embryo with neural folds. (b) Drawing of the human embryo, Stage 10 (week 4), with eight somites showing partial fusion of neural folds to form the neural tube with rostral and caudal neuropores.

Fig. I-4. Drawing of the human embryo, Stage 11 (week 4), with the closing rostral neuropore, two pairs of branchial arches, the heart prominence, body stalk, and widely open caudal neuropore.

Fig. I-5. Drawing of the human embryo, Stage 12 (week 5), diagrammatically represented with the forebrain prominence, three pairs of branchial arches, the upper limb bud, and developing tail. The otic pits are visible.

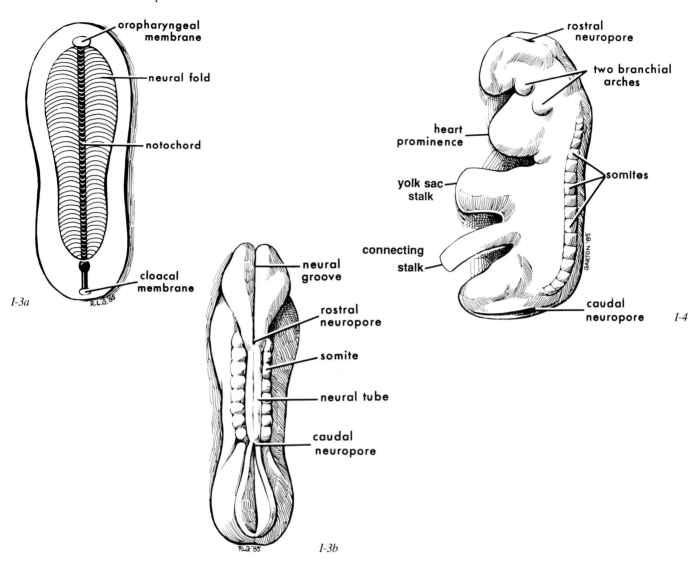

I-3a

oropharyngeal membrane

neural fold

notochord

cloacal membrane

R.L.G.'85

neural groove

rostral neuropore

somite

neural tube

caudal neuropore

RLG'85   I-3b

rostral neuropore

two branchial arches

heart prominence

yolk sac stalk

somites

connecting stalk

GARTON '85

caudal neuropore   I-4

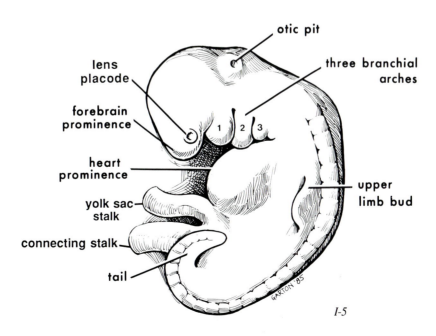

otic pit

lens placode

three branchial arches

forebrain prominence

heart prominence

yolk sac stalk

upper limb bud

connecting stalk

tail

GARTON '85

I-5

The Fifth Week of Development
(Stages 13–15)

The embryo now measures 5 to 10 mm in length. Changes in body form seen during this week are minor, compared to those that occurred during the fourth week, and are characterized by rapid head growth. This extensive head growth is caused mainly by the rapid development of the brain and leads to a further increase in embryonic curvature. As a result, the face is in close contact with the heart prominence. The fourth pair of branchial arches and the lower limb bud are present during Stage 13, which corresponds to approximately 28 to 32 days of development (Fig. I-6a,b).

Lens pits that indicate the future lenses of the eyes are visible on the sides of the head during Stage 14. Elongation with tapering of upper limb buds and the presence of lens pits and nasal pits are the main external features of Stage 14 embryo.

The upper limbs begin to show regional differentiation as the hand plates develop toward the end of the fifth week (Fig. I-6c,d). At this time, the embryo shows other features of Stage 15 such as the appearance of nasal pits, closed lens vesicles, and branchial arches.

Fig. I-6. (a) Schematic drawing of the human embryo, Stage 13 (week 5), showing the presence of all four branchial arches, the lens placode, and otic pit. Note that the lower limb bud is recognizable. (b) Embryo, Stage 13, in the chorionic sac shows a well-preserved embryonic body curvature. Note the four branchial arches, upper and lower limb buds (arrows), and heart prominence (H). The neural tube is completely closed. The yolk sac is labeled Y. (c) Lens vesicle and hand plate formation are prominent features of the Stage 15 embryo (week 5) in this schematic drawing. (d) A well-preserved fresh embryo, Stage 15, showing the lens vesicle with a faint outline of retinal pigment (arrow). The upper limb bud reveals regional differentiation and hand plate formation; body stalk, B; yolk sac, Y.

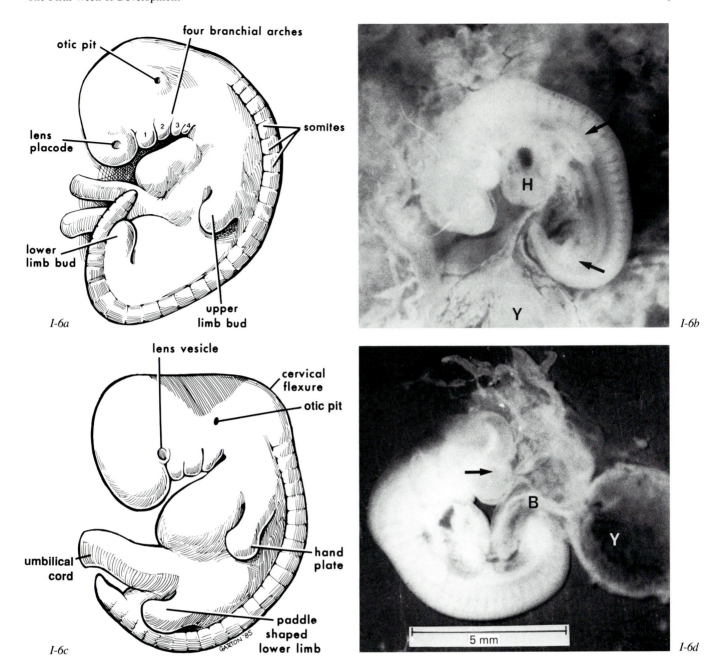

otic pit

four branchial arches

lens placode

1 2 3 4

somites

lower limb bud

upper limb bud

I-6a

H

Y

I-6b

lens vesicle

cervical flexure

otic pit

umbilical cord

hand plate

paddle shaped lower limb

GARTON '85

I-6c

B

Y

5 mm

I-6d

The Sixth Week of Development (Stages 16–17)

The CR length of the embryo in this time period is approximately 10 to 14 mm. The main external features of Stage 16 can be summarized as follows: Nasal pits face ventrally, retinal pigment becomes visible, auricular hillocks appear, and the foot plate is formed.

During Stage 17, embryos are still C shaped, even though the trunk has begun to straighten. The development of finger rays is one of the main hallmarks of this stage, while the formation of basic facial structures advances dramatically. As the medial nasal prominences and maxillary prominences merge the upper lip appears. The nostrils become clearly defined and the eyes are directed more anteriorly (Fig. 1-7a,b,c).

The Seventh Week of Development (Stages 18–19)

At the end of the seventh week, embryos attain a CR length of 20 mm. The head continues to enlarge rapidly and the trunk straightens further. During Stage 18, the elbow region can be recognized on the upper limbs and toe rays appear on the lower limbs (Fig. I-8). In addition, the eyelids are formed and the nipples can be seen.

Stage 19 is characterized externally by trunk elongation, with the result that the head no longer forms a right angle with the back of the embryo. The toe rays are more prominent, but interdigital notches have not yet appeared on the footplate. Physiologic herniation of the intestinal tract into the umbilical cord occurs; these intestinal loops, however, normally "return" to the abdomen by the end of the 10th week.

Fig. I-7. (a) Stage 17 embryo (week 6), with a pigmented eye and auricular hillocks, is shown diagrammatically on lateral view. (b) The nostril and upper lip formation are depicted on front view. The finger rays and the footplate represent other hallmarks of this stage. (c) A fresh, well-preserved embryo, Stage 17, shows trunk straightening and visible somites in the lumbosacral region. The pigmented eye has developed. Digital rays are visible in upper limb buds. Lower limb buds show footplate development.

Fig. I-8. A fresh, well-preserved embryo, Stage 18, has a piece of amnion (A) and chorion (C) attached to the umbilical cord. Note the degenerating yolk sac (Y). Digital and toe rays are discernible, and there are notches between the toe finger rays. The elbow region is appearing.

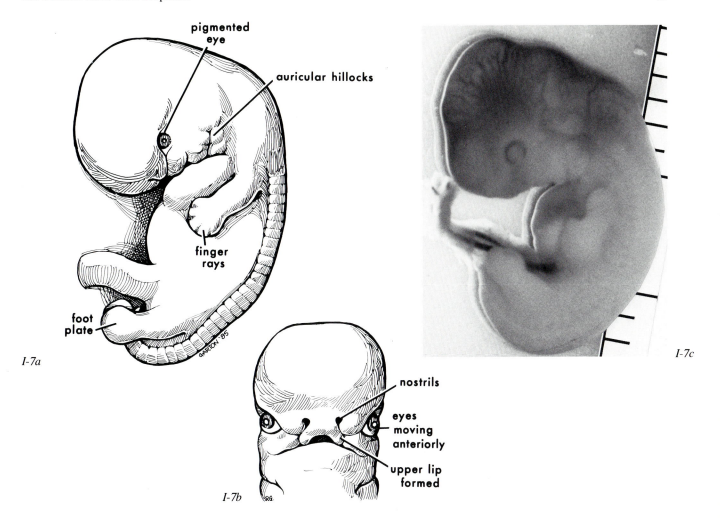

I-7a

I-7b

I-7c

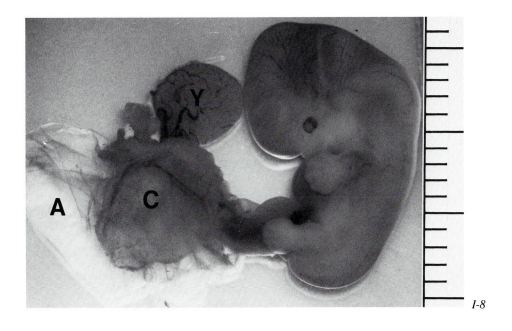

I-8

The Eighth Week of Development
(Stages 20–23)

At the beginning of the eighth week, the fingers are distinct but still webbed. There are notches between the toe rays, and a delicate scalp vascular plexus appears. The edge of the plexus is approximately halfway between the eye–ear level and the vertex of the head (Fig. I-9a,b). Towards the end of the week, the fingers become free and longer and the development of the feet approaches that of the hands. The head becomes more rounded and shows typical human characteristics. The embryo measures 20 mm from crown to rump at the beginning of the week and 30 mm at the end of the week (Fig. I-10a,b).

For more detailed descriptions and information about internal organ development, the reader is referred to O'Rahilly and Muller's *Developmental Stages in Human Embryos*, *Gasser's Atlas of Human Embryos*, and to such comprehensive textbooks as Hamilton, Boyd, and Mossman's *Human Embryology*, Patten's *Human Embryology*, and Moore's *The Developing Human*.

Fig. I-9. (a) Diagram of a human embryo, Stage 20 (week 8), showing distinct fingers still webbed, notches between toe rays and prominent scalp vascular plexus. The elbow is now bent. (b) A fresh, well-preserved embryo showing all the features of Stage 20. However, the scalp vascular plexus is obscured by a generalized vascular congestion. Focal areas of hemorrhage are seen in both upper and lower limbs and the trunk. Arrows point to localized subepidermal edema and focal damaged area in neck and back.

Fig. I-10. (a) Diagram of a human embryo, Stage 23 (week 8), emphasizing the completed development of the face, hands, and feet. Note the persistence of umbilical herniation of some loops of the small bowel. (b) A fresh, well-preserved embryo, Stages 22–23, measures 28 mm crown to rump length. Note the developing and fusing eyelids. The external ear is well developed (arrow); the toes are free and longer. Note the scalp vascular plexus (arrow) and the umbilical cord (U).

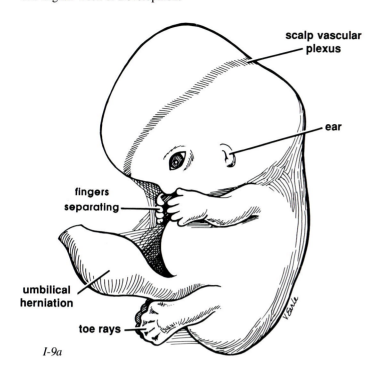

scalp vascular plexus

ear

fingers separating

umbilical herniation

toe rays

I-9a

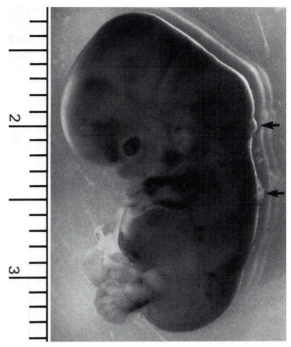
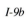

I-9b

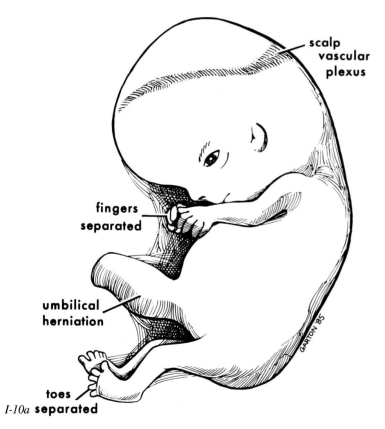

scalp vascular plexus

fingers separated

umbilical herniation

toes separated

I-10a

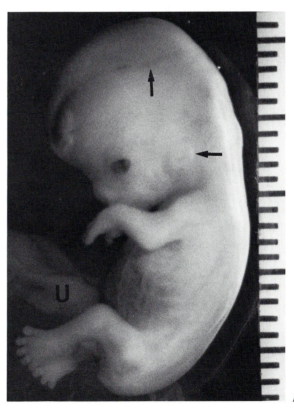

U

I-10b

References

Crowley LV: *An Introduction to Clinical Embryology*, Chicago, Year Book Medical Publishers Inc., 1974.

Gasser RF: Atlas of Human Embryos, Hagerstown, Harper and Row, 1985.

Hamilton, WJ, Boyd JD, Mossman MW: *Human Embryology*, ed 4, Baltimore, MD, Williams & Wilkins Co., 1978.

Kalousek, DK: Confined chorionic mosaicism in human gestations, in Fraccaro M, Simoni B, Brambati B (eds). *First Trimester Fetal Diagnosis*, Springer, Berlin, 1985, pp 130–136.

Keibel F, Mall FP: *Manual* of *Human Embryology*, Philadelphia, Lon-don, Lippincott, 1910, vol I; 1912, vol II.

Mall FP: On stages in the development of human embryos from 2 to 25 mm long. *Anat Anz* 46:78–84, 1914.

Markert CL, Petters RM: Manufactured hexaparental mice show that adults are derived from three embryonic cells. *Science* 202:56–58, 1978.

Moore KL: *The Developing Human. Clinically Oriented Embryology*, ed 3, Philadelphia, Saunders, 1982.

O'Rahilly R, Muller F: *Developmental Stages in Human Embryos*, Washington, DC, Carnegie Institution, Publication 637, 1987.

Patten BM: *Human Embryology*, ed 3, New York, McGraw-Hill, 1968.

Streeter GL: *Developmental Horizons in Human Embryos*, Washing-ton, DC, Carnegie Institute of Embryology, 1951.

CHAPTER II

Previable Fetal and Placental Development

Fetal Development (9–18 weeks)

No formal system of staging exists for the fetal period. Development during the whole fetal period (9 weeks to term) primarily concerns rapid body growth and further differentiation of organs and tissues. There are no dramatic changes in the external appearance and, therefore, greater emphasis is placed on crown–rump (CR) and crown–heel (CH) measurements to establish fetal developmental age (see Appendix II, Table II-2). The fetal period can be subdivided into the previable fetal period (9 to 18 weeks of development) and the viable fetal period (19 to 38 weeks of development). Between the 9th and the 18th week, the rate of body growth is very rapid. The CR length of the fetus increases from 30 to 180 mm. The weight of the previable fetus varies and is unreliable as an indicator of developmental age (Golbus and Berry, 1977).

Ultrasound measurements of CR length closely correlate with the CR measurements obtained from aborted fetuses. Ultrasound measurements are predictive of fetal gestation age with an accuracy of ± 3 days at 10 weeks to ± 2 weeks at 20 weeks. Assessment of fetal growth by ultrasound can be improved by measuring the biparietal diameter, the circumference of the head, the dimensions of the trunk, and the length of the femur (Nicolaides and Campbell, 1986).

During the previable fetal period, changes in the external appearance of the fetus are subtle but progressive. The head is about one-third the size of the fetal body at 12 weeks, and approximately one-quarter at the 16th week. The lower limb length increases more rapidly compared to the upper limb, which, during the embryonic period, is more developmentally advanced. At 16 weeks, both forearms and legs have increased in length, crossed the midline, and overlapped each other. The fingers are flexed. The marked cervical flexure present in the embryo is lost by the 12th week. The spine is straight with a mild dorsal flexure.

The most obvious hallmarks of previable fetal development are summarized below and illustrated in Figs. II-1–II-12.

During the *9th week*, the eyes are closing or closed. The head occupies almost one half the fetus. The legs are short and the thighs are relatively small. The external genitalia are not yet distinguishable as male or female. Some intestinal coils are still herniated into the proximal end of the umbilical cord. The *tenth week* is characterized by the "return" of the intestine into the abdomen. During the *11th* and *12th week*, the external genitalia of male and female fetuses are distinguishable and the neck is well defined. The fingernails are clearly developed in the *13th week*. Lower limb development catches up with upper limb growth by the *14th week*. Eyebrows and scalp hair become visible and the ears stand out at the end of the *16th week*. During the *17th* and *18th week*, the skin becomes covered with a mixture of a fatty secretion from the fetal sebaceous glands and desquamated epidermal cells; this is called the *vernix caseosa*. Brown fat starts to form during this time in the perirenal area, posterior sternum, and neck area around the subclavian and carotid vessels.

At week 9 the external genitalia of the two sexes are similar in their appearance. There is a phallus with urethral groove, urogenital folds and labio-scrotal swellings (Fig. II-11a).

By 11–12 weeks in the male the phallus develops into the penis. The urogenital folds fuse with each other along the ventral surface of the penis to produce a median penile raphe over the urethra. Hypospadias result from incomplete fusion of the urogenital folds. The penile urethra forms when an ectodermal ingrowth at the tip of the glans occurs. The labio-scrotal swellings fuse in the midline to form the scrotal raphe (Fig. II-11b,e).

In the female the phallus develops into the clitoris. The urogenital folds do not fuse and they form the labia minora and the labio-scrotal swellings form the labia majora. Although a primitive urethral groove forms it regresses (Fig. II-11c,d).

Three palatal processes develop to separate the nasal cavity and the mouth: median palatine process (the primary palate)

15

and two lateral palatine processes (the secondary palate). They form between weeks 5–12.

The primary palate develops at the end of the fifth week and in the formed hard palate it represents only the very small part anterior to the incisive foramen.

The secondary palate is the primodium of the hard and soft palates extending from the region of the incisive foramen posteriorly. The secondary palate develops from 2 horizontal mesodermal projections that extend from the internal aspects of the maxillary prominences. These projections approach each other and fuse in the midline. They also fuse with the primary palate and the nasal septum. The fusion between the nasal septum and the palatine processes begins anteriorly during the ninth week and is completed posteriorly in the region of the uvula by the twelfth week (Fig. II-12a,b).

Various techniques are available for assessing the status of the fetus and for diagnosing certain diseases and developmental abnormalities before birth. These include ultrasound examination, chorionic villus sampling, amniocentesis, fetal blood sampling, and fetoscopy. The principles of these techniques and their application are summarized in Appendix I.

Functional maturation of individual organs begins in the early fetal stage and approaches completion at about the 36th week of pregnancy. Detailed information on the development and maturation of individual systems can be found in embryology textbooks (Hamilton et al., 1978; Moore, 1982). A brief summary of selected organs maturation is given below.

Heart

The anatomy of the fetal heart is identical to that of the newborn throughout the whole fetal period. Histologically, cardiac muscle is cross-striated and easily identifiable. Purkinje's cells of the conducting system become noticeable in early fetal hearts as bundles of muscle cells with relatively fewer fibrils of larger diameter than the rest of the cardiac muscle cells. They occur mainly under the endocardium and extend without interruption from the atrium to the ventricle.

Lungs

In the early fetus, the pulmonary lobes and fissures are well established. Pulmonary parenchyma development can be divided into three stages—pseudoglandular, canalicular, and terminal sac phase. Only the pseudoglandular and canalicular stages are present during the early fetal period. In the *pseudoglandular period (5–15 weeks)*, the lung is a loose mass of connective tissue with actively proliferating bronchi, the walls of which are lined with tall columnar nonciliated epithelial cells, which may be pseudostratified. Capillaries are sparse and not in direct contact with the epithelial cells. During the *canalicular period (16–22 weeks)*, the lung becomes highly vascular and the epithelial cells of the developing bronchi become ciliated and lose their pseudostratification.

Goblet cells producing mucus are found in bronchial surface epithelium from 11 weeks. Mucus-producing glands in the submucosa first appear in the trachea; around the 11th to 12th week, they appear in the bronchi. Complete tracheal rings are formed by 10 weeks; the cartilage in bronchi at 16 weeks. Irregular breathing movements start around 12 weeks and become regular by the 18th week of development.

Alimentary Tract

The epithelium of the mucous membrane of the alimentary tract, although completely derived from endoderm, shows variable differentiation. The esophagus, during early fetal life, is lined by columnar cells many of which are ciliated. Later, these cells are gradually replaced by stratified squamous epithelium. In the stomach, the first glandular pits are seen at 6 weeks and extend over the whole stomach mucosa by 10 weeks. At 11 weeks, differentiation of the parietal cells begins, and at 12 to 13 weeks, the chief cells and mucous neck cells differentiate. Differentiation of the various types of secretory and absorptive cells in the small and large intestine occurs in early fetal life. The splanchnic mesoderm of the primitive gut differentiates to form, first, the inner circular layer of the musculature (4–9 weeks) and, then, the outer longitudinal muscle (6–11 weeks). The muscularis mucosae appears after 12 weeks. Peristalsis occurs in the isolated fetal gut as early as the 11th week of development. At 10 weeks, ganglia are readily seen in the myenteric plexus.

Liver

At about 8 to 9 weeks, the liver represents 10% of the body weight due to its rapid growth and erythroblast accumulation. During the early fetal stage, the basic glandular unit

---

Fig. II-1. Normal fetus week 9—(a) anterior and (b) lateral view. Note relatively large head sizes. As the body straightens, the head is better defined. The eyelids are fused. A small loop of intestines is still herniated into the umbilical cord (arrow).

Fig. II-2. Normal fetus week 10—(a) anterior and (b) lateral view. The thin skin allows easy visualization of underlying blood vessels. The intestine has returned into the abdomen.

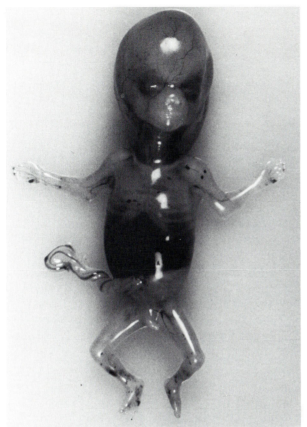

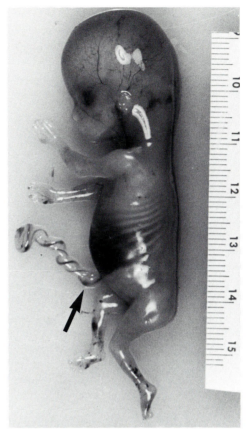

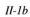

II-1a

II-1b

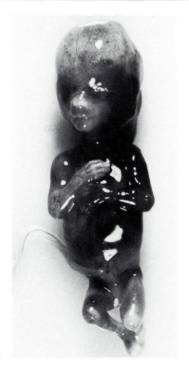

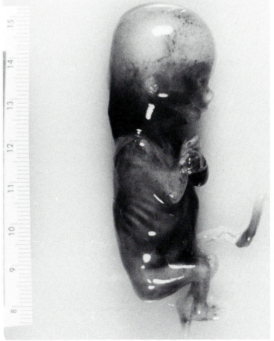

II-2a

II-2b

of the liver, seen through childhood and adulthood, is established. This unit, called the *hepatic triad*, consists of the bile ducts, hepatic artery, and portal vein. Differentiating biliary ducts can be seen in the connective tissue at 9 to 12 weeks. Extramedullary hematopoiesis is prominent in hepatic mesoderm throughout the whole early fetal period.

Pancreas

During the fetal period, branching of the original endodermal outgrowth that gave rise to the pancreas continues in the form of solid epithelial sprouts that become canalized to form the collecting ducts (10 weeks). The acini arise by sprouting from the tips of collecting ducts. After 16 weeks, secretory granules appear in the acinar cells, which coincides with the release of pancreatic secretion into the intestinal lumen.

In the 10th to the 11th week of fetal life, the endocrine cells of the islets of Langerhans develop from small groups of cells with a dark cytoplasm, which appear initially among the clear epithelial cells of the ducts and subsequently bud into the surrounding stroma. Islet α and β cells can be distinguished in these islets from the beginning. This process of budding off from the duct wall continues throughout the fetal period and islets can be found at various stages of development and size.

Kidney

The kidney develops from the nephrogenic blastema and ureteric bud. The nephrogenic blastema gives rise to the nephrons each consisting of a glomerulus and a proximal convoluted tubule, a loop of Henle, and a distal convoluted tubule. The ureteric bud differentiates into collecting tubules, renal pelvis, calyces, and ureter. Glomeruli are first formed in the region of the metanephric tissue that, in the definitive kidney, constitutes the juxtamedullary region. It has been estimated that approximately 20% of nephrons are morphologically formed and mature at 9 to 11 weeks of development, and another 10% is added at 14 to 18 weeks. By 12 weeks, the kidney is differentiated into a cortex and a medulla. By 16 weeks, development of the pyramids is advanced. Glomeruli continue to form from the metanephric blastemal cap until about 36 weeks of gestation.

Ovary

The primordial germ cells pass to the female gonad during embryonic development. After 10 weeks, the ovary can be histologically identified. Its structure is characterized by small groups of cells forming primordial ovarian follicles that result from the fragmentation of the sex cords.

Testis

The testis can first be histologically identified in embryos of about 17 mm CR length (41 days), when the male gonadal blastema is subdivided into cords by developing fibrous tissue bundles. The *tunica albuginea*, the outside dense fibrous layer, forms at the end of the embryonic period (week 8). Primordial germ cells are incorporated into the sex cords which then become canalized to form the *seminiferous tubules*. The interstitial *Leydig cells* are prominent from 12 to 20 weeks of gestation. They are derived from the mesenchymal cells of the stroma.

Adrenal Gland

The adrenal gland consists of a mesodermal cortex and a neuroectodermal medulla. Both the cortex and medulla are functional at an early fetal age. Fetal adrenals are relatively large. At four months, the glands are larger than the fetal kidney. The great size is due to the extensive development of the fetal cortex, which constitutes about 80% of the fetal gland.

Thymus

The glandular structure of the thymus develops as the epithelial mass and becomes surrounded by a mesenchymal condensation at 9 weeks of development. At 10 weeks, a lobular pattern is established after vascular invasion. At 11 weeks, the thymic medulla and cortex can be distinguished, and Hassall's corpuscles develop as aggregates of large cells with granular eosinophilic cytoplasm.

Fig. II-3. Normal fetus week 11—(a) anterior and (b) lateral view. Differentiation of the external genitalia is completed.

Fig. II-4. Normal fetus week 12—(a) anterior and (b) lateral view. The vessels under the skin are still prominent. The external genitalia are easily distinguishable. This fetus is male. The external ear is well differentiated.

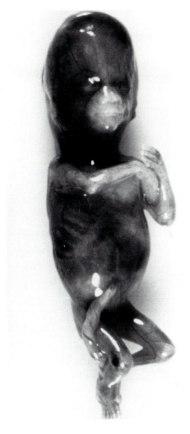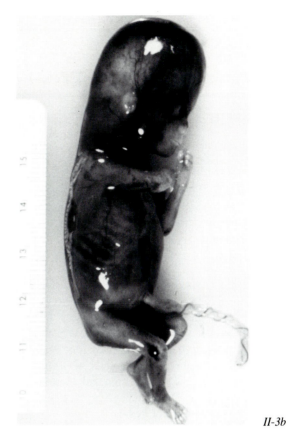

II-3a   *II-3b*

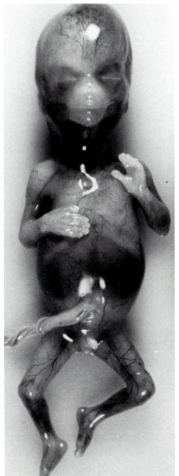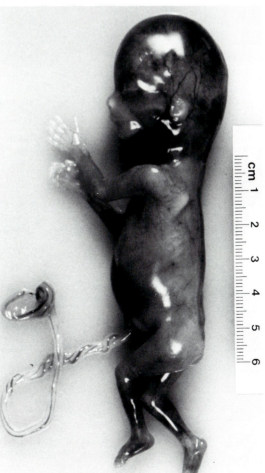

II-4a   *II-4b*

Thyroid

Differentiation, with follicle formation, occurs between 8 and 11 weeks of gestation. Between 12 and 18 weeks, the function of the hypothalamic/ pituitary/thyroid axis is established.

Skin

Hair follicles are seen in the skin by 12 weeks and have become more abundant by 18 weeks. Epidermal ridges are established in the hands by 17 weeks.

Placental Development

The placenta develops into a circumscribed and discrete organ from about the 10th gestational week. There is no clear demarcation between the embryonic and fetal stages of placental development but rather there is a gradual maturation of villi in the area of implantation, and loss of function of those villi not involved in the formation of the mature organ.

Up to about the 8th week, villi cover the entire surface of the chorionic sac. As the sac grows, the villi facing the uterine cavity lose their blood supply and degenerate to give rise to the *chorion laeve*. At the same time, the villi associated with the decidua basalis proliferate and branch rapidly giving rise to the *chorionic plate* and the chorionic villi of the placenta. The placental shape is usually discoid. As a result of villous invasion of maternal decidua, the surface of the placenta is divided into 10 to 30 irregular convex areas—lobules or *cotyledons*. Each cotyledon represents the proliferation of two or more main stem villi and their many branches. The cotyledons are separated by decidual tissue wedges.

The placental membranes are formed by a fusion of the chorion laeve and the amniotic sac at about 9 weeks of development. Fusion before 9 weeks is abnormal and characteristic of embryonic growth disorganization. Delayed fusion or no fusion may be seen in the amnion rupture sequence and limb-body wall syndrome when the extraembryonic coelom between the chorion and the amnion persists (see Chapter VI).

Amniotic fluid is secreted by the amniotic cells and is also derived from the maternal blood by transport across the amnion and by fetal secretion of urine. Its volume increases slowly. There is about 30 ml at 10 weeks, 350 ml at 20 weeks, and 1000 ml by 37 weeks. Radioactive isotope studies have shown that the water in the amniotic fluid changes every three hours, with large volumes of fluid moving via the placental membranes. Some fluid is directly absorbed into the fetal circulation from the fetal gastrointestinal and respiratory systems. About 98% water, amniotic fluid contains protein, carbohydrates, fats, enzymes, hormones, and pigments. The number of desquamated fetal epithelial cells increases as pregnancy progresses. Amniotic fluid is important to the development of the embryo and fetus since it cushions the embryo/fetus against injuries and allows free movement.

The *umbilical cord* develops from the connecting stalk, which is extraembryonic mesoderm, joining the caudal end of the embryonic disc and primary yolk sac to the internal surface of the chorion. As the tail of the embryo is formed and the embryo grows, the connecting stalk becomes attached to the ventral surface of the embryo and contains the vitelline duct (communication between the yolk sac and the midgut of the embryo), and the allantoic diverticulum accompanied by the allantoic vessels (two umbilical arteries and two umbilical veins, although only one of the latter persists). The mature umbilical cord consists of two umbilical arteries and one vein within the mesodermal core of loose mesenchyme. Because the umbilical vessels are longer than the cord, twisting and bending of the vessels is common. The cord is covered by amniotic epithelium and may contain remnants of the allantoic diverticulum and the vitelline duct. The embryonic umbilical cord is at first only a few millimeters long, but, as the gestational sac and the embryo grow, it increases its length rapidly (Appendix II, Table II-5). At 14 weeks, the average length of the umbilical cord is 16 cm. At full term, it is normally about 50 to 54 cm (Hamilton et al., 1978).

Fig. II-5. Normal fetus week 13—(a) anterior and (b) lateral view. Note the progressive growth of the lower extremities.

Fig. II-6. Normal fetus week 14—(a) anterior and (b) lateral view. Relative micrognathia is a normal finding at this stage of development. The lower limbs are equal in size to the upper limbs.

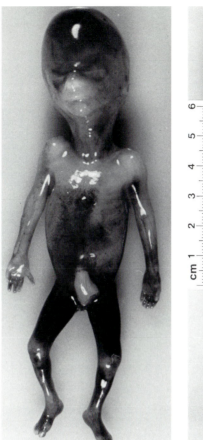

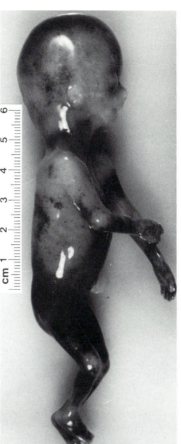

II-5a   *II-5b*

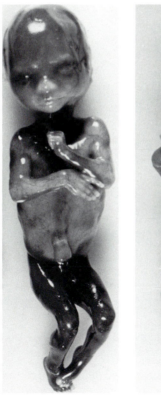

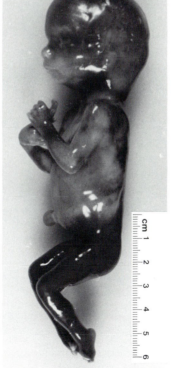

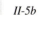

II-6a   *II-6b*

Fig. II-7. Normal fetus week 15–(a) anterior and (b) lateral view. On lateral view, the partially opened mouth gives the false impression of severe micrognathia.

Fig. II-8. Normal fetus week 16–(a) anterior and (b) lateral view. The final relative proportions of femur to tibia/fibula are attained.

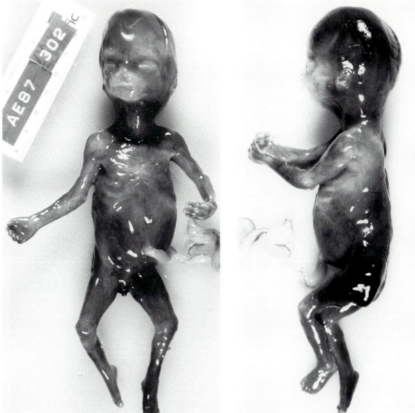

II-7a   *II-7b*

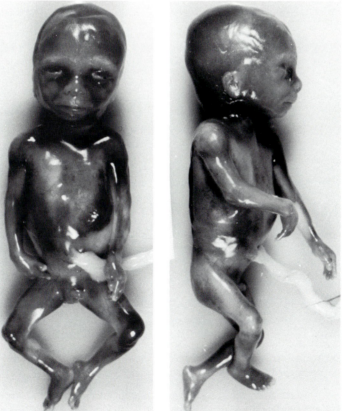

II-8a   *II-8b*

Fig. II-9. Normal fetus week 17−(a) anterior and (b) lateral view. Epidermal ridges used for dermatoglyphics studies are established.

Fig. II-10. Normal fetus week 18−(a) anterior and (b) lateral view. The eyebrows are well developed, and both the fingernails and toenails are defined. The external ear is differentiated.

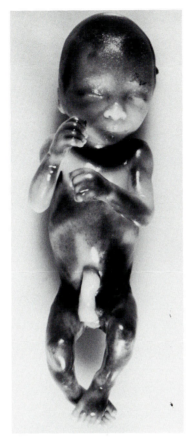

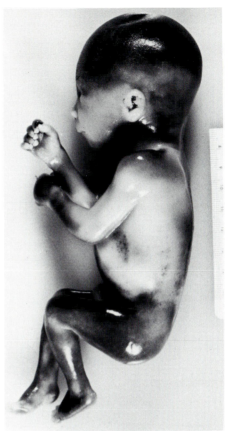

II-9a

II-9b

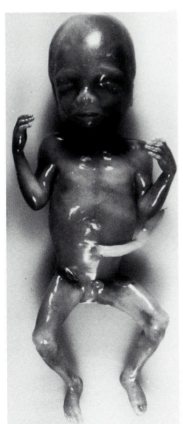

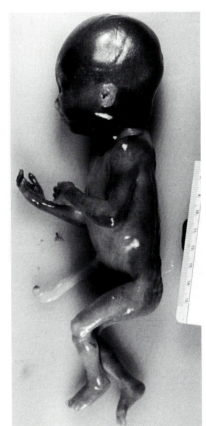

II-10a

II-10b

Fig. II-11. (a) A nine-week-old fetus. Close up: undifferentiated external genitalia. Arrows indicate the phallus, labioscrotal swellings, and anus. (b) A fourteen-week-old fetus with normal male genitalia. Arrows indicate the umbilical cord, penis, and anus. (c) A fourteen-week-old fetus with normal female genitalia. Arrows indicate the umbilical cord, clitoris, and anus. (d) Eighteen-week-old fetus with normal female genitalia. Arrows indicate the umbilical cord, clitoris, and anus. (e) Eighteen-week-old fetus with normal male genitalia. Arrows indicate umbilical cord, penis, and anus.

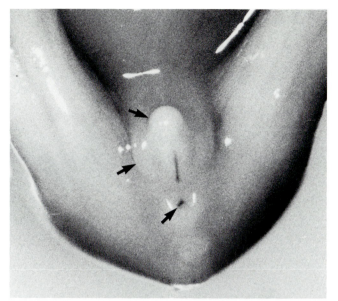

II-11a

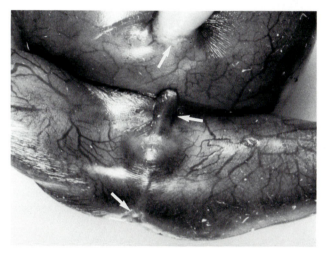

II-11b

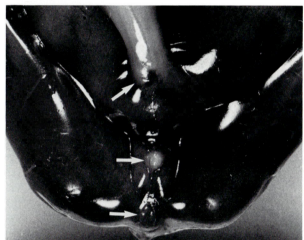

II-11c

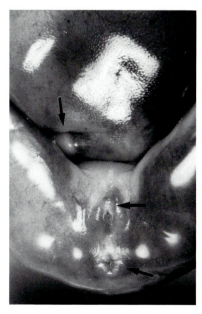

II-11d

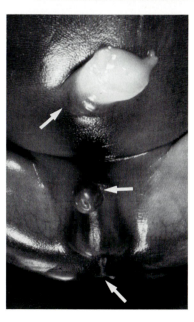

II-11e

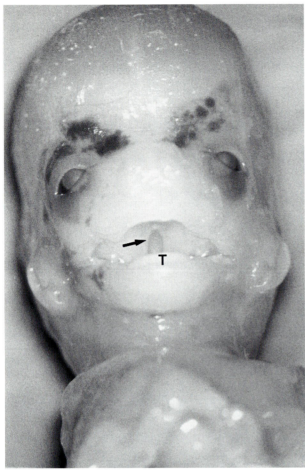

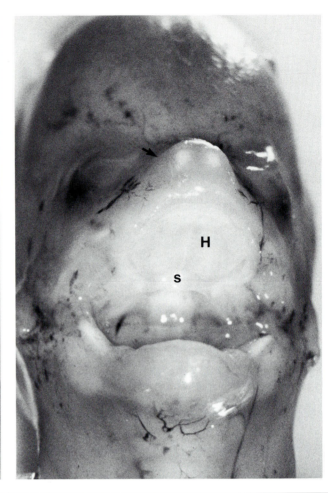

II-12a   *II-12b*

Fig. II-12. (a) Nine-week-old fetus with well-formed upper lip and physiologically partially fused hard and completely opened soft palate (arrow); tongue, T. (b) Completely closed hard (H) and soft (S) palate; 14-week-old fetus. Arrow points to nose.

References

Golbus MS, Berry LC Jr: Human fetal development between 90 and 170 days post menses. *Teratology* 15:103–108, 1977.

Hamilton WJ, Boyd JD, Mossman MW: *Human Embryology*, ed 4, Baltimore, MD, Williams & Wilkins Co, 1978.

Moore KL: *The Developing Human. Clinically Oriented Embryology*, ed 3, Philadelphia, Saunders Co, 1982

Nicolaides KM, Campbell S: *Diagnosis of Fetal Abnormalities by Ultrasound*. ed 2, Milunsky A (ed): *Genetic Disorders and the Fetus*, Plenum Press, New York, London, pp 521–570, 1986.

B. Abortion and Specimen Examination

CHAPTER III

Abortion

Definitions Used in the Study of Abortions

The term *conceptus* (*products of conception*) includes all the structures that develop from the zygote: the embryo, or fetus, and the placenta with its membranes. The developing human is considered to be an *embryo* from conception until the end of the eighth week, by which time all major organ systems have been formed. From the beginning of the ninth week until birth, the developing human is called a *fetus*.

Abortion is defined as the premature expulsion or removal of the conceptus from the uterus before it is able to sustain life on its own. In this book, 18 developmental weeks (20 gestational weeks) is considered the lower limit of viability. An older fetus can be delivered either stillborn or as a premature, mature and postmature newborn.

A *threatened abortion* is characterized by bloody discharge from the pregnant uterus without cervical dilation, whereas an *inevitable abortion* is associated with profuse or prolonged bleeding with cervical dilation or effacement. An *incomplete abortion* means that some of the presumably dead conceptus has not yet passed; if a dead conceptus is retained for at least four weeks, the term used is *missed abortion*. *Recurrent* (*repeated*) *abortion* is defined as three or more spontaneous abortions.

An *induced abortion* or *therapeutic abortion* or *termination of pregnancy* may be performed because the mother's health is in jeopardy or for a wide variety of social reasons, which include rape, incest, government policy concerning family size, undesired pregnancy, or a defective fetus. As yet, there is no general term that specifically refers to an induced abortion performed because the fetus is found to be abnormal on prenatal diagnosis.

The duration of intrauterine development can be described by several different terms. The *developmental* or *conceptional age* of an embryo and fetus extends from the day of fertiliza-
tion to the day of intrauterine death or expulsion of the live conceptus. In contrast, *gestational* or *menstrual age* extends from the first day of the last menstrual period to the expulsion or removal of the conceptus. Therefore, gestational age is 2 weeks greater than developmental age.

The *intrauterine retention period* refers to the time between the death of the embryo/fetus and its expulsion or removal.

The *early spontaneous abortion* occurs in the embryonic period, up to the end of the eighth developmental week. The *late spontaneous abortion* refers to death in the 9th to 18th week of fetal development.

Terms Related to Developmental Abnormalities

Efforts have been made to classify developmental defects according to their pathogenesis. The definitions of terms related to embryonic and fetal developmental abnormalities presented here are based on the report of an International Working Group (Spranger et al., 1982).

A *malformation* refers to a morphological defect resulting from an intrinsically abnormal developmental process in the embryo, such as an open neural tube defect, a cleft palate, or an organ agenesis. It is important not to diagnose a malformation in a conceptus too young to have developed the particular organ or tissue. A *disruption* results from the extrinsically caused breakdown of, or interference with, an originally normal developmental process such as might occur as the result of local mechanical pressure by amniotic bands, which for example, amputate a limb or limbs. A *deformation* means an abnormal form, shape, or position of the fetus caused by such mechanical constraints as fetal compression due to oligohydramnios. A *developmental dysplasia* refers to an abnormal organization of cells into tissue(s) and the morphological result(s) of this abnormality. Dysplasias can be *generalized* (osteogenesis imperfecta) or *localized* (hemangioma).

Relationships between multiple anomalies in the same fetus also have special terms that attempt to reflect etiologic or pathogenetic concepts. A *developmental field*, a term borrowed from experimental embryology, refers to a region of the embryo that reacts as a spatially coordinated developmental unit. A defect of a developmental field implies its disturbance to such a degree that it cannot repair itself and so produces several malformations in this region. A *sequence* refers to multiple anomalies derived from a single cause: thus, an obstructive uropathy sequence is initiated by a urinary outflow obstruction and produces oligohydramnios, fetal compression, and deformations. A *syndrome* is a pattern of multiple anomalies thought to be pathogenetically related. Although often implying a known single cause or underlying defect, the term *syndrome* implies less knowledge of the pathogenesis of the anomalies themselves than does the term sequence. Finally, an *association* refers to multiple anomalies that appear to be nonrandom in occurrence and are not known to be a field defect, a sequence, or a syndrome, such as the VATER association (Vertebral defects, Anal atresia, T-E fistula, Renal and Radial defects).

Our current knowledge of etiology and pathogenesis of specific conditions varies widely. By definition, we know the pathogenesis of deformations and disruptions but usually not the etiologies; the same applies to the constellations of anomalies that are defined as sequences. In contrast, etiology is better understood than pathogenesis in some malformations and syndromes. There are numerous situations, however, in which neither pathogenesis nor etiology is clear.

Classifications of Spontaneous Abortions

Every spontaneous abortus should be examined in the pathology laboratory, not only to confirm that it is, in fact, a "product of conception" but also to determine the presence of absence of embryonic/fetal defect and to ascertain the cause of embryonic/fetal death so that informative and accurate counseling of the parents can be initiated.

Classifications of the final pathological diagnosis on abortuses facilitate our monitoring of human reproductive loss on a larger scale. Of the many anatomic and pathologic classifications of spontaneous abortuses, two different types are illustrated here.

The classification of Fujikura et al. (1966)—based on gross examination of 353 early and late abortuses, excluding hydatidiform moles and ectopic pregnancies—follows:

Group I   Incomplete specimen
Group II   Ruptured empty sac
                a) with cord stump
                b) without cord stump
Group III Intact empty sac
Group IV   Embryo or fetus present with or without a chorionic sac or placenta
                a) normal embryo or fetus
                b) abnormal embryo, including nodular, amorphous, and cylindrical embryos
                c) embryo or fetus with focal anomalies
                d) unable to determine normality

Rushton (1984) examined 814 abortuses, including hydatidiform moles. His classification, which is particularly useful in classifying specimens without a grossly evident embryo or fetus, is based on microscopic placental morphology, as follows:

Group 1   Early conceptions (mean developmental age, 9.4 weeks)
                Most villi show microscopic hydropic change
                Most villi show stromal fibrosis with vascular obliteration
                Intermediate between the above changes, with about equal proportions of hydropic villi and stromal fibrotic villi.
Group 2   Conceptions with macerated embryos/fetuses (mean developmental age, 14.1 weeks)
                Normal/abnormal embryo or fetus may be present or absent
                Collapsed villous vessels that may contain degenerated nucleated red cells and be impregnated with iron and calcium salts
                Obliterative fibrosis of vessels with collagenization of villous stroma
                Deposition of iron and calcium salts on trophoblastic basement membrane and within villous stroma
                Perivillous and intervillous fibrin deposition starting on the maternal surface and progressing toward the fetal surface
Group 3   Conceptions with nonmacerated fetuses (mean developmental, age 18.6 weeks)
                Normal/abnormal fetus may be present
                More likely than Group 2 to show evidence of chorioamnionitis and retroplacental hemorrhage.

Mechanisms of Spontaneous Abortions

Although much is known about the important components in the development and maintenance of conception, such as the trophoblast, uterus, corpus luteum, and fetal and maternal circulation, the mechanism of many spontaneous abortions is poorly understood.

About 50% of spontaneous abortions are associated with chromosome abnormalities such as trisomy and triploidy. About 95% of these conceptuses die in the first trimester. In order to understand why death occurred it becomes necessary to focus on the systems needed to keep the fetus alive, such as the placenta and, in particular, the trophoblast. Perhaps most chromosomally abnormal embryos and fetuses die because the trophoblast, which is fetal tissue, is not functioning normally. Kalousek et al. (1989) found that the trophoblast of the few trisomy 13 and 18 fetuses who survive to birth is not completely trisomic but rather mosaic, that is, it also contains a normal cell line with 46 chromosomes. This suggests that an abnormal non-mosaic trophoblast is responsible for the early lethality of the majority of trisomy 13 and 18 conceptions.

Failures of fetal and maternal circulations are less common causes of spontaneous abortions than are trophoblast malfunctions. Intrauterine fetal death due to umbilical cord constrictions by amniotic bands (Kalousek and Bamford, 1988) or premature placental separation are obvious but relatively rare examples of such circulatory failure prior to 20 weeks of gestation.

Intrauterine infection is a common cause of second trimester pregnancy loss.

It is an interesting empirical observation that fetuses with severe malformations such as complex congenital heart defects, large abdominal wall defects, or neural tube defects generally proceed to term if they are not detected prenatally. There is not yet an explanation for the relatively high rate of spontaneous abortion of some minor developmental defects such as cleft palate or localized limb abnormalities, (Poland et al., 1981).

In the natural history of a spontaneous abortion, it is common for the embryo or fetus to die some time prior to its expulsion from the uterus. The interval between death and expulsion may be from one to eight weeks. Therefore in evaluating the conceptus, it is important to distinguish between those changes that occurred before embryonic/fetal death and those that occurred after death. The most obvious consequence of prolonged intrauterine retention is maceration or autolysis of the embryo/fetus. No maceration occurs in the chorionic sac or the placenta because they are continuously nourished via the maternal circulation. After embryonic/fetal death, the principal changes within the chorionic villi are atrophy of the cytotrophoblast, clumping of nuclei in the syncytial trophoblast, fibrosis of villous stroma, and collapse of villous vessels (Chapter X).

Frequency of Spontaneous Abortion

The highest conceptus mortality occurs in the earliest weeks of pregnancy, usually before a woman realizes that she is pregnant (Kline and Stein, 1985). In vitro fertilization studies show that only 40% of embryos have the capacity to implant; and up to 23% of implantation failures can be attributed to embryonic nonviability and some 30% to maternal factors (Yovich, 1985). Other studies have been based on repetitive pregnancy testing of women who might conceive. One such study reports that 43% of the conceptions aborted before 20 weeks and that about 33% of the conceptions had been diagnosed only by beta-subunit hCG pregnancy testing (Miller et al., 1980). Another found that 62% of the conceptuses were lost prior to 12 weeks, with most losses occurring subclinically (Edmonds et al., 1982). A recent study indicates that the total rate of pregnancy loss after implantation, including clinically recognized spontaneous abortion, is 31% (Wilcox et al., 1988). Clearly, these are only estimates, since the beta-subunit hCG pregnancy test may not be positive until the blastocyst implants at about seven days postfertilization.

Many reports in the literature indicate that some 15 to 20% of *clinically recognized* pregnancies spontaneously abort in the first and second trimester (Glass and Golbus, 1984). A similar figure was obtained from a prospective study of more than 30,000 pregnant women, which showed an estimated probability of spontaneous abortion of 14.4% between weeks 5 and 28 of gestation (Harlap and Ramcharan, 1980).

The frequency of embryonic loss in the 1st trimester and of previable fetal loss in the 2nd trimester is difficult to establish, since most clinical studies do not subdivide first and second trimester losses based on the development of the conceptus (Harlap and Ramcharan, 1980) and many dead embryos are retained until second trimester.

Etiology of Spontaneous Abortion

Chromosomal Abnormalities

Approximately 50% of all spontaneous abortions are chromosomally abnormal, with the four main classes of abnormality being trisomy (27%), polyploidy (10%), sex chromosome monosomy (9%), and structural rearrangements (2%). About half of the abnormal karyotypes that occur in first trimester abortions are various forms of autosomal trisomy, of which trisomy 16 is the most frequent; it accounts for about one third of all trisomies. Trisomy of chromosomes 21 and 22 are the next most frequent cause and account for a further 20% of all trisomies. Trisomies 5, 11, 17, and 19 are very rare, and trisomy 1 has only been observed in the preimplantation embryo (Watt et al., 1987). It is not yet clear whether the variation in numbers of trisomies involving different chromosomes reflects the frequency of their occurrence in gametes or their relative preimplantation lethality (Jacobs and Hassold, 1987).

During the previable fetal period, the reported prevalence of chromosomal abnormalities is between 4 and 44% when gestational age is used to evaluate fetal development. How-

mosaicism in trophoblast and intrauterine survival of trisomies 13 and 18. *Am J Hum Genet* 44:338–343, 1989.

Kline J, Stein Z: Very early pregnancy, in Dixon RL (ed): *Reproductive Toxicology*, New York, Raven Press, 1985, pp 251–265.

Miller JF, Williamson E, Glue J, Gordon YB, Grudzinskas JG, Sykes A: Fetal loss after implantation. A prospective study. *Lancet* 2: 554–556, 1980.

Mowbray JF: Success and failures of immunization for recurrent spontaneous abortion, in Beard RW, Sharp F (eds): *Early Pregnancy Loss*, Springer-Verlag, pp 325–336, 1988.

Naeye RL, Tafari N: *Risk Factors in Pregnancy and Diseases of the Fetus and Newborn*; Baltimore, MD, Williams & Wilkins, p 194, 1983.

Poland BJ, Miller JR, Harris M, Livingston J: Spontaneous abortion: A study of 1961 women and their conceptuses. *Acta Obstet Gynecol Scand* (suppl 102):5–32, 1981.

Robertson WB, Brosens I, Dixon HG: The pathological response of the vessels of the placental bed to hypertensive pregnancy. *J Pathol Bacteriol* 93:581–592, 1967.

Roman E, Stevenson AC: Spontaneous abortion, in Barron SL, Thomson AM (eds): *Obstetrical Epidemiology*. London, Academic Press, 1983, pp 61–87.

Rushton DI: The classification and mechanisms of spontaneous abortion. *Perspect Pediatr Pathol* 8:269–286, 1984.

Shepard TH: *Catalog of Teratogenic Agents*, ed 5. Baltimore, MD, Johns Hopkins University Press, 1986.

Smithells RW, Sheppard S, Schorah CJ, Seller MJ, Nevin NC, Harris R, Read AP: Possible prevention of neural tube defects by preconceptional vitamin supplementation. *Lancet* 1:339–340, 1980.

Spranger J, Benirschke K, Hall JG, Lenz W, Lowry RB, Opitz JM, Pinsky L, Schwarzacher HG, Smith DW: Errors in morphogenesis: Concepts and terms. Recommendations of an International Working Group. *J Pediatr* 100:160–165, 1982.

Syrop CH, Varner MW: Systemic lupus erythematosus. *Clin Obstet Gynecol* 26:547–557, 1983.

Thomas ML, Harger JH, Wagener DK, Rabin BS, Gill TJ: HLA sharing and spontaneous abortion in humans. *Am J Obstet Gynecol* 151:1053–1062, 1985.

Watt JL, Templeton AA, Messini I, Bell L, Cunningham P, Duncan RO: Trisomy 1 in an eight cell human pre-embryo. *J Med Genet* 24:60–64, 1987.

Weitkamp LR, Schachter BZ: Transferrin and HLA. Spontaneous abortion, neural tube defects, and natural selection. *N Engl J Med* 313: 925–929, 1985.

Yovich JL: Embryo quality and pregnancy rates in in-vitro fertilization. *Lancet* i:283–284, 1985.

Wilcox AJ, Weinberg CR, O'Connor JF, Baird DD, Schlatterer JP, Canfield RE, Armstrong EG, Nisula BC: Incidence of early loss of pregnancy. *New Engl J Med* 319:189–194, 1988.

CHAPTER IV

Principles of Early Abortion Specimen Examination

For accurate pathologic evaluation of the early aborted conceptus, all aborted tissues and a thorough obstetrical, medical, and family history are required. The need for complete clinical information is similar to that required for other types of intrauterine death. Menstrual dates are valuable for dating the gestational sac and embryo. Information about drug ingestion (e.g., anticonvulsive medication) or exposure to infection during pregnancy (e.g., rubella) is essential for directing the pathologist's attention to a specific problem and for proper handling of the specimen. A history of previous reproductive failures or a family history of a particular congenital, morphological, or metabolic defect may significantly influence the investigative approach. An example of a consultation request form is given in Appendix II (Table II-7).

The aborted tissue should be submitted fresh, not fixed in formalin, in a sterile, or at least a clean, tightly closed container or bag so it does not dry out. Small specimens should be kept moist with gauze soaked in sterile saline. An example of instructions for mailing aborted tissue is given in Appendix II (Table II-8).

An early spontaneous abortus is best examined in a large sterile Petri dish, with sterile instruments, under a dissecting microscope. Sterile technique allows the taking of samples for tissue culture and chromosome analysis, if indicated, after the examination under the dissecting microscope is completed. The dissecting microscope should have a camera attachment so that photographic documentation can supplement the gross description. When a small embryo is identified, after its position in the sac has been recorded and a photograph taken, it is best transferred to a smaller sterile dish for further examination. Since embryonic specimens are generally fragile, it is recommended that they be examined floating in saline or after fixation.

There are basically two types of early abortion specimens: complete and incomplete. A *complete specimen* of early abortion consists of an intact chorionic sac, which may be empty or may contain various embryonic or extraembryonic tissues (see below). Decidual tissue and blood clots are usually present. Often the chorionic sac is ruptured or, following uterine curettage, fragmented. Careful examination of all submitted material for the presence of an embryo should be done in such cases, since the embryo may be present outside the ruptured chorionic sac or among curettings. When an embryo is not found, an opened chorionic sac is categorized as an *incomplete specimen*. In many instances, only chorionic villi, decidua, and blood clots are available for pathologic examination (Fig. IV-1).

Not infrequently, the specimen contains just decidua and blood clots. Confirming the presence of an intrauterine implantation site in endometrial curettings is important to exclude ectopic pregnancy (O'Connor and Kurman, 1988).

Examination of the Chorionic Sac

Intact Chorionic Sac

An intact chorionic sac is commonly found as a fluctuant globular structure in a pear-shaped specimen that represents a decidual cast of the uterine cavity (Fig. IV-2a-c). Such specimens should be carefully opened from the narrow end to release the chorionic sac intact. Smaller intact chorionic sacs may be received free, not embedded in decidua, and surrounded only by blood clots. The chorionic sac varies from 10 to 80 mm in diameter. The suface of a well-developed chorionic sac is usually completely covered by abundant chorionic villi (Fig. IV-3a). Sparse villous development (Fig. IV-3b) or no villous development (Fig. IV-3c) is usually seen in sacs showing also abnormal development of amnion, yolk sac and embryo.

After opening the intact chorionic sac, the presence or absence of amniotic sac, yolk sac, body stalk/cord, and embryo should be noted (Fig. IV-3d). When the amniotic sac is present, its size and relationship to the chorionic sac must be recorded. An abnormally large amniotic sac and its premature fusion with chorion are the most frequent abnormalities (Fig. IV-3e). Aberrant amniotic sac development, in the form of cysts, also has been reported (see Chapter X). Recording an abnormal size and/or position of the yolk sac allows further insight into the sequence and timing of the insult during early embryogenesis. Examination of the embryo is described below.

Villi are best observed in saline under the dissecting microscope. Normal villi are of uniform diameter, with a symmetrical branching appearance and multiple buds along their length (Fig. IV-4a). Sparse development and abnormal morphology (swelling, clubbing, and hypoplasia) of chorionic villi are common in early abortion specimens. Villi with swollen tips are described as clubbed (Fig. IV-4b), villi with clear vesicles at their end are as cystic (Fig. IV-4c), and villi with few buds or thin irregular branches as hypoplastic (Fig. IV-4d). Histologically, clubbed and cystic villi are usually hydropic and avascular. Hypoplastic villi are fibrotic, with vascular obliteration.

Fig. IV-1. Incomplete specimen consisting of decidua (D), blood clots (B), and fragments of chorionic sac (C).

Fig. IV-2. Examples of decidual casts. (a) Intact decidual cast of the uterine cavity; arrow, bulging chorionic sac. (b) Opened decidual cast with chorionic sac in place; arrow, exposed chorionic sac. (c) Decidual cast with ruptured chorionic sac (arrow).

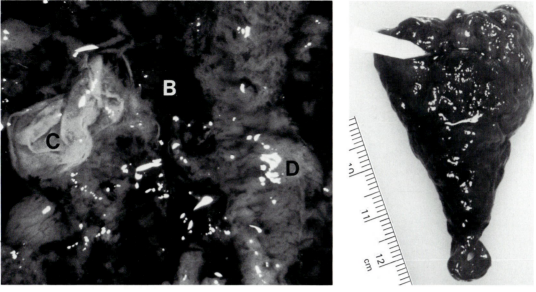

IV-1

IV-2a

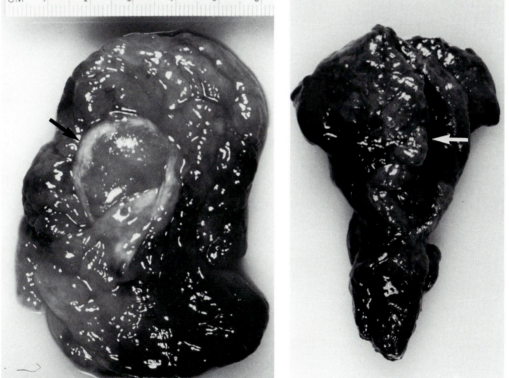

IV-2b

IV-2c

Fig. IV-3. Different types of intact chorionic sacs. (a) A small intact chorionic sac, 1.7 cm, with abundant, well-developed villi. (b) Intact 1.8-cm chorionic sac, with sparse villous development. (c) Intact empty chorionic sac, 2.5 cm in diameter, with hardly any villous development. (d) Intact amniotic sac with an embryo (Stage 17). Note yolk sac (arrow) and a space (S) between the amniotic sac and the opened chorionic sac. (e) Intact chorionic and amniotic sacs containing bloody amniotic fluid and an embryo (Stage 20). Arrow points to retinal pigment. Note the sparse chorionic villi. The amnion and chorion are prematurely fused.

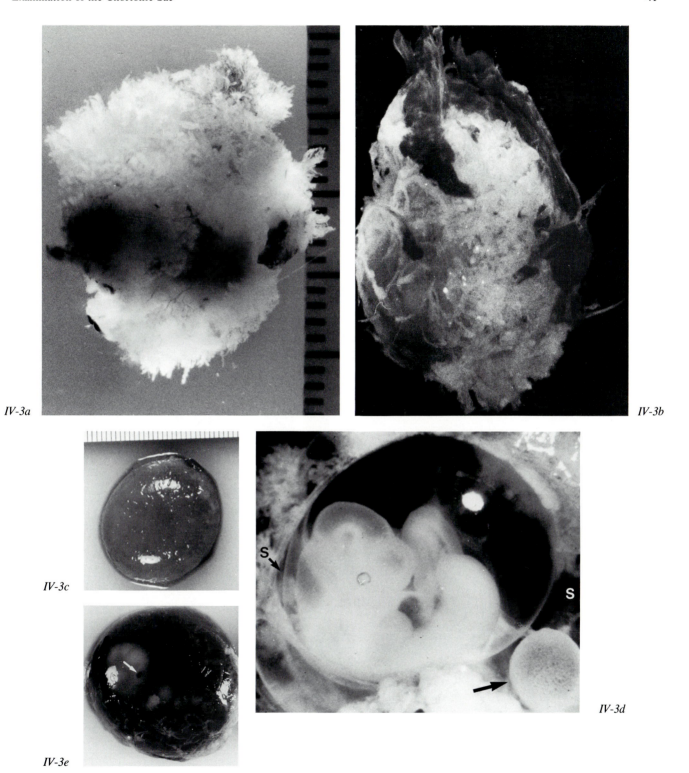

IV-3a

IV-3b

IV-3c

IV-3e

IV-3d

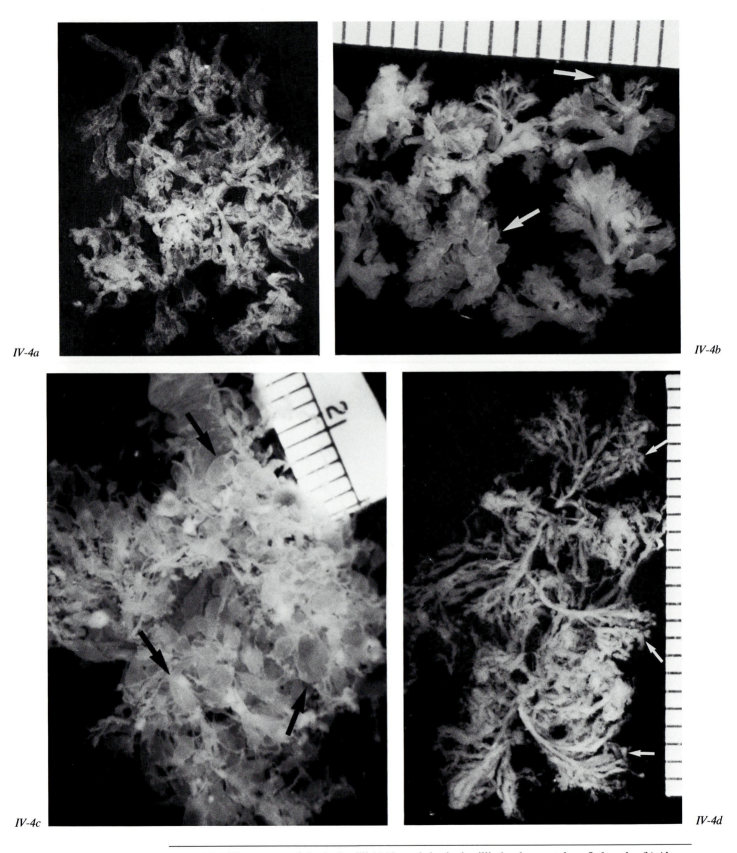

IV-4a

IV-4b

IV-4c

IV-4d

Fig. IV-4. Different types of chorionic villi (a) Normal chorionic villi, developmental age 5–6 weeks. (b) Abnormal clubbed (arrow) chorionic villi, developmental age 6–8 weeks. (c) Abnormal villi showing focal cystic dilation (arrows). (d) Abnormal villi showing marked stromal fibrosis and villous clubbing (arrows).

Ruptured Chorionic Sac

A ruptured chorionic sac has a collapsed corrugated appearance due to amniotic fluid loss. The embryo is frequently missing from such a sac (Fig. IV-5). Even in the absence of the embryo, evaluation of the presence or absence of the amniotic sac, its size and relationship to the chorion, the presence of the body stalk and yolk sac, together with a histological examination of the villi allow categorization of the specimen as a normally or an abnormally developing gestational sac.

Fragmented Chorionic Sac

A fragmented chorionic sac without a detectable embryo can yield information about embryonic development only if the villi are examined histologically (Fig. IV-6). Histological abnormalities in the chorionic villi relate to the time at which embryogenesis was disturbed. If embryonic death occurred before the embryonic circulation was established in the placental villi, that is, before the end of the third week, the villi will be avascular and hydropic and will have attenuated trophoblast layers. However, if the embryonic circulation was established, and then ceased because of embryonic death, increased villous stromal cellularity, followed by fibrosis, and vascular obliteration will be seen (Rushton, 1984).

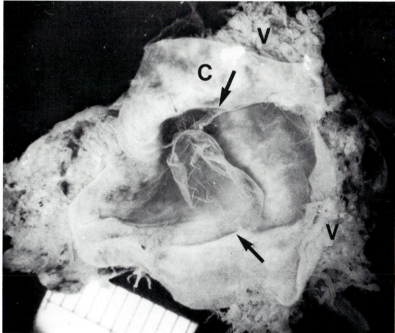
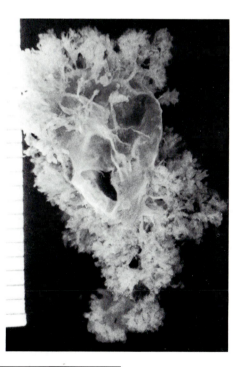

IV-5 *IV-6*

Fig. IV-5. Ruptured chorionic sac (C) with well-developed villi (V) and amniotic sac with focal attachments (arrows). No embryo and yolk sac can be identified.

Fig. IV-6. Ruptured chorionic sac. No embryo, yolk sac, or amnion can be identified.

Retained Chorionic Sac

After embryonic death, the primary changes within the chorionic villi are atrophy of the cytotrophoblast, clumping of nuclei in the syncytial trophoblast, fibrosis of villous stroma, and collapse of villous vessels. A further change is an increase in villous fluid content, which is usually described as hydropic degeneration in clubbed or cystic villi. Villous swelling tends to be patchy. More diffuse hydropic degeneration, resembling a hydatidiform mole but without trophoblastic abnormalities, may be associated with retained chromosomal trisomies and triploidies with two sets of paternal chromosomes. Calcifications in villi either focal or along basement membrane are common.

Examination of the Embryo

Early experience with the pathologic examination of aborted human embryos has been summarized by Mall in several publications (Mall, 1907, 1908, 1917; Mall and Meyer, 1921). Mall observed that embryonic developmental anomalies are more common than defects at birth (Mall, 1917) and that many embryonic defects are difficult to identify as specific malformations. He called embryos with ill-defined abnormal development stunted or cylindrical embryos (Mall, 1908). The high incidence of abnormal embryos in abortion specimens has been confirmed by many other investigators (Hertig and Sheldon, 1943; Hertig and Rock, 1949; Colvin et al., 1950; Nishimura et al., 1968; Kajii et al., 1980; Poland et al., 1981; Kalousek, 1987). The study of Poland et al. (1981) is one of the largest morphologic studies of early spontaneous abortion. In this study, normal embryos were detected in only 16% of 1126 specimens, whereas abnormal embryos were seen in 84% of these specimens. Among the abnormal embryos, a specific systemic or localized defect(s) in otherwise normally developing embryos occurred in 5%, whereas generalized abnormal embryonic development (see Chapter VI) was reported in 79% of these specimens.

External examination of embryos provides data for determining their *developmental stage*. The examination consists of detailed evaluation of characteristic facial, limb, and body features under the dissecting microscope. The embryonic developmental age is established by correlating crown–rump (CR) length and developmental stage. The difference greater than 14 days between the developmental age thus derived and the gestational age calculated from the last menstrual period reflects the length of retention in utero after embryonic death.

The CR length of the embryo is obviously the single most important measurement. It should be taken without attempting to straighten out normal flexures (Fig. IV-7a,b,c). Since embryos in the third and early fourth weeks are nearly straight, their linear measurement indicates greatest length. In embryos with flexed heads (fifth and sixth weeks of development) the CR length is actually a neck–rump measurement. The true CR length can be measured only in older embryos. Since the length of an embryo is not the only criterion for establishing age, the pathologist should also evaluate the embryo's developmental characteristics. Length and development can then be compared and developmental age established.

Any discrepancy between embryonic length and a specific developmental hallmark points to the existence of a developmental defect. For example, if a fresh, well-preserved embryo measures 5 mm and there is incomplete closure of the rostral neuropore, an open neural tube defect is a likely diagnosis. To evaluate embryonic development accurately, it is essential to have in the laboratory, available for comparison, a set of photographs or drawings of normal human embryos from anterior, posterior, and lateral views, as well as a set of actual fixed embryonic specimens, both of which illustrate the normal development of each stage (O'Rahilly and Muller, 1987).

Although the CR length is very important for staging normally developing embryos and embryos with focal defects, it is meaningless for staging embryos with growth disorganization (see Chapter VI), since such embryos do not follow a normal pattern of development.

Human embryos collected from spontaneously aborted tissues can be grouped into four major categories:

1. Normal embryos—harmoniously developed for their developmental stage (See Chapter I)
2. Growth-disorganized embryos—embryos with highly abnormal embryonic development (See Chapter VI)
3. Embryos with specific developmental defects (See Chapters VI and VIII)
4. Macerated, damaged, unclassifiable embryos

Fig. IV-7. Measuring the embryonic crown–rump length. (a) Fresh embryo (Stage 15) with an attached body stalk, part of the yolk sac, and a portion of the amnion; The arrows indicate how the crown–rump length should be measured. (b) A degenerated embryo (Stage 13) lacking the normal embryonic curvature. This specimen demonstrates the difficulty in measuring the crown–rump length of degenerated specimens. (c) Crown–rump length in advanced embryo (Stage 23) is measured the same way it is done in fetuses.

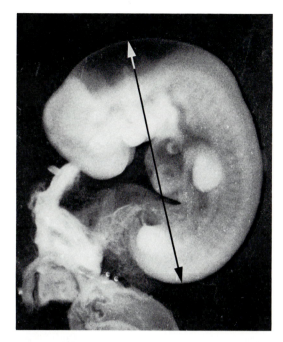

IV-7a

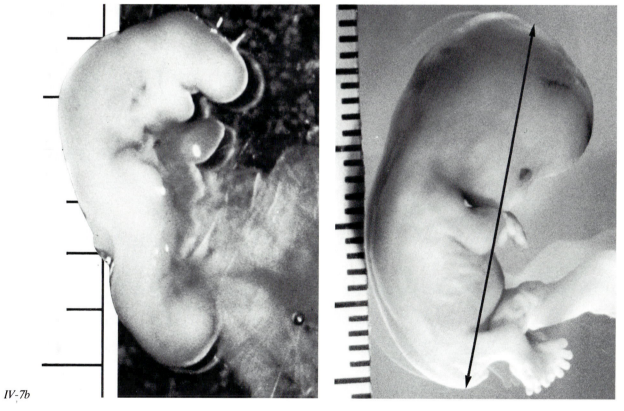

IV-7b

IV-7c

Damaged and severely macerated embryos cannot be properly evaluated (Fig. IV-8a,b,c). Their developmental age can be estimated, based on specific structure or organ development (e.g., hand, eye), but developmental defects cannot be diagnosed, since maceration alone can mimic such focal defects as the open neural tube defect or cleft lip. The difficulty in evaluating retained embryonic specimens has been recognized by Streeter (1930), who estimated that, on average, embryonic retention is as long as six weeks. Although ultrasound examination can detect intrauterine embryonic death, the number of observed macerated embryonic conceptions has not been reduced as most pregnancies are screened by ultrasound in the second trimester.

Fig. IV-8. Damaged and degenerated embryos. (a) Severely fragmented embryo (approximately Stage 18) (see upper limb bud, L); arrows, brain, eye, and cord. (b) Abnormal embryo in two fragments showing facial clefting (arrow), delayed limb bud development (L), and cystic umbilical cord (C). (c) Abnormal triploid embryo with damaged neck area and lower segment of the body. The umbilical cord is cystic (C).

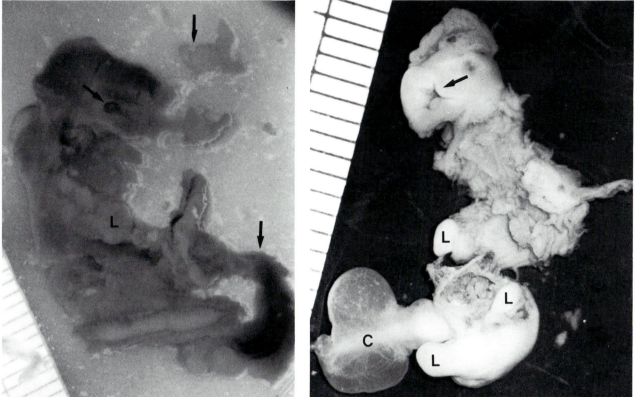

IV-8a

IV-8b

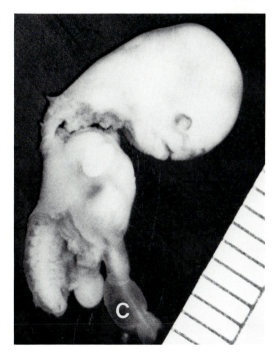

IV-8c

References

Colvin ED, Bartholomew RA, Grimes WH, Fish JS: Salvage possibilities in threatened abortion. *Am J Obstet Gynecol* 59:1208–1224, 1950.

Hertig AT, Rock J: A series of potentially abortive ova recovered from fertile women prior to the first missed menstrual period. *Am J Obstet Gynecol* 58:968–993, 1949.

Hertig AT, Sheldon WH: Minimal criteria required to prove prima facie case of traumatic abortion or miscarriage. *Ann Surg* 117:596–606, 1943.

Kajii T, Ferrier A, Niikawa N, Takahara H, Ohama K, Avirachan S: Anatomic and chromosomal anomalies in 639 spontaneous abortuses. *Hum Genet* 55:87–98, 1980.

Kalousek DK: Anatomic and chromosome anomalies in specimens of early spontaneous abortion. Seven year experience, in Gilbert EF, Opitz JM (eds): *Genetic Aspects of Developmental Pathology*, New York: Alan R. Liss Inc., for the National Foundation–March of Dimes BD: OAS JXXIII (1), 1987, pp 153–168.

Mall FP: On measuring human embryos. *Anat Rec* 6:129–140, 1907.

Mall FP: A study of the causes underlying the origin of human monsters. *J Morphol* 19:3–368, 1908.

Mall FP: On stages in the development of human embryos from 2 to 25 mm long. *Anat Anz* 46:78–84, 1914.

Mall FP: On the frequency of localized anomalies in human embryos and infants at birth. *Am J Anat* 22:49–72, 1917.

Mall FP, Meyer AW: Studies on abortuses: A survey of pathologic ova in the Carnegie embryological collection. *Embryol Carnegie Inst* 12:1–364, 1921.

O'Connor DM, Kurman RJ: Immediate trophoblast in uterine curretings in the diagnosis of ectopic pregnancy. *Obstet Gynecol* 72:665–670, 1988.

O'Rahilly R, Muller F: *Developmental Stages of Human Embryos*, Washington, DC, Carnegie Institution, Publication 637, 1987.

Nishimura M, Takano K, Tanimura T, Yasuda M: Normal and abnormal development of human embryos. *Teratology* 1:281–290, 1968.

Poland BJ, Miller JR, Harris M, Livingston J: Spontaneous abortion: A study of 1961 women and their conceptuses. *Acta Obstet Gynecol Scand* (suppl 102):5–32, 1981.

Rushton DI: The classification and mechanisms of spontaneous abortion. *Perspect Pediatr Pathol* 8:269–286, 1984.

Streeter GL: Focal deficiencies in fetal tissues and their relation to intra-uterine amputation. *Contr Embryol Carnegie Inst* 22:1–44, 1930.

CHAPTER V

Principles of Late Abortion Specimen Examination

Late abortion specimens, 9 to 18 developmental weeks or 11 to 20 gestational weeks, consist of an identifiable fetus and a placenta and each can be examined separately. Again, it is essential that the obstetrical history be available to the pathologist. Both fetus and placenta should be submitted fresh, and without fixation, as quickly as possible to the pathology department so that cytogenetic, microbiological, or biochemical studies can be initiated when required. If immediate transport is not possible, then the fetus and placenta should be refrigerated in a sterile, dry, tightly closed container. Fixation should be used only if refrigeration is not available and if several days' delay in delivery to pathology is anticipated. In such cases, a small piece of fetal skin and a segment of the placenta, including the villi, the chorion, and the amnion, should be separately submitted in tissue culture media.

Examination of the Fetus

Routine examination of the fetus consists of both external and internal examinations, radiologic examination, photographic documentation, and histologic examination.

External Examination

The fetus should be weighed and measurements of crown–rump (CR) length, crown–heel (CH) length, and head circumference should be recorded. The CR length is the main criteria used for establishing the fetal developmental age (see Appendix II, Table II-2). Tables are also available for determining developmental age from foot and hand lengths (see Appendix II, Table II-3). These can be used instead of the CR length when the specimen is incomplete or fragmented (Fig. V-1), or they can be used in addition to the CR length to verify its accuracy.

A detailed external examination of the fetus is an essential part of the morphologic studies. Careful inspection of the face to determine if abnormalities of the eyes, nose, mouth, palate, mandible, and ears are present should be made; it should be remembered that some specific features and some facial characteristics of common syndromes, such as trisomy 21 or trisomy 18, may be only partially developed or even absent in previable fetuses (Fantel et al., 1980). The shape of the head, the position of the ears, and the presence or absence of scalp hair should be noted. In the examination of the limbs, the length, the number of digits and their position, and presence or absence of flexion deformities are equally important. An example of a protocol for recording the external examination findings is given in Appendix II (Table II-9).

Macerated and damaged fetuses should not be ignored, even though they may appear to be grossly distorted (Fig. V-2,3a). In spite of molding and distortion, such external malformations as neural tube defect, cleft lip and palate, syndactyly, polydactyly, amputations, and constrictions can be easily diagnosed. Artifacts produced by maceration in previable fetuses are different from those seen in embryos (see below). It is essential for diagnosis of amniotic rupture sequence that small amputations of digits or constrictions of the umbilical cord by a thin amniotic band are noted on external examination of the retained macerated fetus. Otherwise, the cause of intrauterine death due to cord constriction by an amniotic band may be missed (Chapter VI-12).

The external examination and the internal examination of nonmacerated fetuses are usually done in a fresh state. However, macerated fetuses should be fixed prior to internal dissection, since their tissues are fragile and artifacts may easily be introduced.

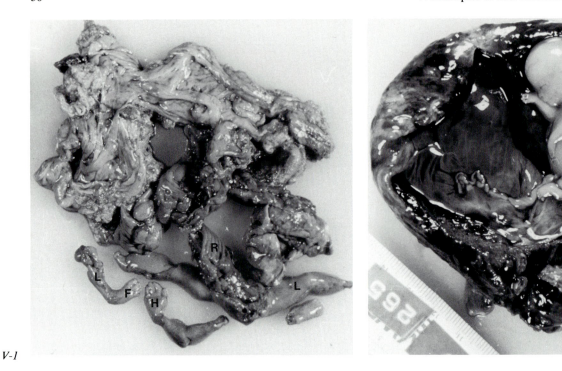

Fig. V-1. Specimen after cervical dilation and curettage for removal of a dead fetus. Note the rib cage (R), legs (L), hand (H), and foot (F).

Fig. V-2. A macerated retained fetus (12 developmental weeks) inside an amniotic and chorionic sac. Note that the amnion and chorion are now closely apposed; arrow, partially peeled amnion.

Fig. V-3. (a) A macerated, fixed, 13-week fetus with marked distortion of the facial structures and limbs. In spite of the distortion, such developmental anomalies as the small mandible, small mouth, and large head can be diagnosed. (b) A 15-week female fetus with sloughing skin, relaxed jaws but no damage to body wall. (c) A severely macerated, 17-week male fetus, with collapsed skull and thorax. Note the sunken eyes and the artifactual elongation of the neck and the low set ears. (d) A macerated, formaldehyde-fixed, 17-week fetus. Note the shrinkage of the skin.

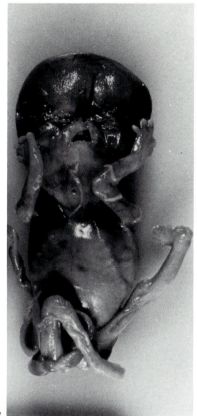

V-3a

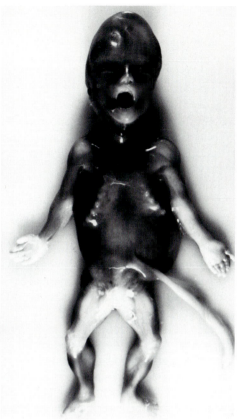

V-3b

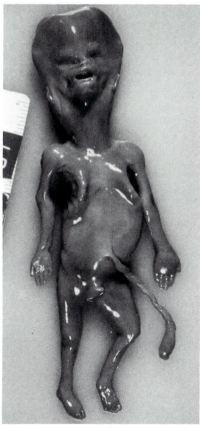

V-3c

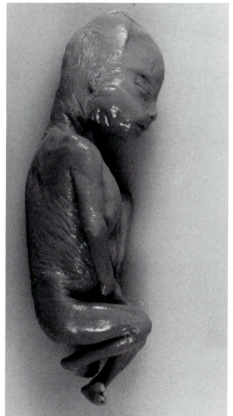

V-3d

Internal Examination

Dissection is usually done in the manner of a mini-autopsy (Fig. V-5). It may be helpful to secure the fetal limbs on a corkboard. Smaller fetuses (9–11 weeks) can also be examined with the dissecting microscope after slicing the trunk at 0.5- to 1-cm intervals (Berry, 1980). The internal examination should not be directed only toward the diagnosis of such obvious abnormalities as organ agenesis, a diaphragmatic hernia, malrotation of intestine, or a cleft palate. Data on palatal closure in early previable fetuses is shown in Appendix II (Table II-4). Meticulous dissection, identical to that of the perinatal autopsy technique, should identify all internal malformations, including congenital heart defects. The use of a magnifying lens or a dissecting microscope is especially recommended for examination of the fetal heart. An example of a protocol for recording the internal examination findings is given in Appendix II (II-9). In cases in which abnormal morphogenesis has been identified on external examination, the incidence of internal developmental defects is high; the likelihood of finding a major internal malformation, however, is only 2% if no external malformations are present (Rushton, 1981). All internal organs should be weighed and the weight compared to normal values to estimate developmental age (Tanimura et al., 1971). If the weight has not been established, it is not possible to diagnose organ hypoplasia.

Examination of the brain is feasible only in nonmacerated fetuses. The brain is usually completely liquified in macerated fetuses. Brain tissue should be removed after fixation in situ, with a widely open skull, in 10% formaldehyde or Bouin fixative for at least a week (Fig. V-6). Precautions to avoid damage of immature brain tissue must be followed (Isaacson, 1984). The examination of the brain not only allows the diagnosis of such specific developmental defects as hydrocephalus or agenesis of the corpus callosum, it is also particularly important in any case of suspected symmetric intrauterine growth retardation (see Chapter VI).

Artifacts

Artifactual abnormalities are frequently found in fetuses that are either spontaneously aborted or terminated in the second trimester of pregnancy (Knowles, 1986).

A common artifact, the tearing of skin and muscle, is due to delivery trauma (Fig. V-4a). It can occur anywhere in the fetal body, but it is most frequent in the abdominal, thoracic, and neck areas. The traumatic nature of the defect is usually obvious in the thorax and neck, but confusion with developmental defects of abdominal wall closure—gastroschisis and omphalocele—can occur when the tear involves the abdominal wall. A careful inspection of the defect, especially its irregular margins, allows its traumatic origin to be identified.

Disruption of such developmental abnormalities as an omphalocele sac or an encephalocele sac requires that the pathologist be familiar with this type of an artifact and direct a search for vestiges of the sac around the circumference of the defect.

Autolysis and degeneration interfere with the evaluation of normal development. In early fetuses, it is difficult to distinguish between opened eyes due to eyelid degeneration and a primary defect in eyelid closure. A similar difficulty arises in the evaluation of the lower lumbar and sacral areas in macerated fetuses (9–11 weeks) when the widening of the spinal canal due to autolysis may mimic an open neural tube defect.

Another artifactual defect seen in macerated retained fetuses is the so-called primitive neuroectodermal tumor (Fig. V-4b,c). This artifact is the result of a squeezing of the brain tissue into the spinal cord and along the spinal nerves into the retroperitoneal and retropleural spaces or the neck area (Kalousek et al., 1988). On gross examination, it resembles an invading tumor; histologically, it is seen as fragmented brain tissue. The finding of this artifact appears to be confined to a developmental age of 9 to 16 weeks, and it may be related to certain developmental characteristics of this period.

Contractures of the limbs, especially contractures without pterygia, are impossible to evaluate on fixed specimens, since they can be produced by the process of fixation.

Fig. V-4. Macerated normal fetuses: (a) A 14.5-week male fetus shows sloughing skin (face, neck, and hands) with a damaged abdominal wall. The fetus is lying on the exposed bowel (arrows); umbilical cord, C. (b) A spontaneously aborted, degenerated, 18.5-week female fetus with a history of a 4-week-long intrauterine retention. Note the extensive tumor-like masses in the retroperitoneal and retropleural space (arrows). (c) A macerated, 16-week female fetus with a 45,X chromosomal complement. Note in the retroperitoneal areas the tumor-like lesions (t), which had bilaterally spread into the inguinal region (arrow).

Fig. V-5. Dissection of a 17-week male fetus with trisomy 21 (perinatal autopsy technique). The thoracic and abdominal cavities are opened for organ removal.

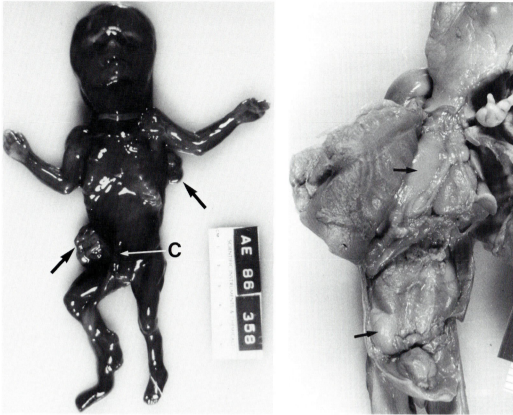

V-4a

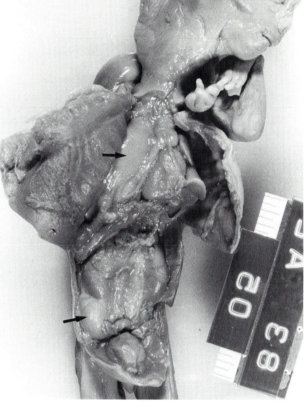

V-4b

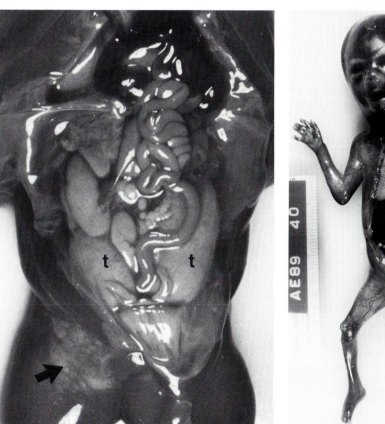

V-4c

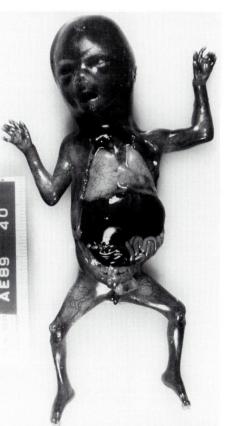

V-5

Equally difficult to evaluate are dysmorphic features in macerated and fixed fetuses. In such specimens, the pathologist must be satisfied with the diagnosis of only clearly defined defects and note that the dysmorphism could not be evaluated due to maceration or to fixation artifacts.

Photographic Documentation

Photographic documentation of all detected developmental defects is mandatory. Photographs of the anterior and lateral aspect of the whole fetus are a useful minimum record (Fig. V-7), but close-ups of all detected malformations should also be taken. Photographs of internal malformations are usually taken under a dissecting microscope to allow a magnified view. The importance of recording fetal abnormalities photographically cannot be overstressed. It identifies the range of abnormalities within a particular syndrome, allows comparisons to be made, and makes reevaluation of the case or evaluation by consultant syndromologists possible.

Radiologic Examination

Morphologic assessment of the abnormal fetus should also routinely include a radiographic examination to determine the developmental age of bone and to document skeletal anomalies. This is best done prior to evisceration, using a Faxitron cabinet or a standard mammography machine. An anterior–posterior (A-P) projection of the whole fetus, which can be conveniently accommodated on an 18 × 24 cm film, is sufficient in most circumstances. If skeletal abnormalities are demonstrated in the A-P projection, then appropriate lateral views and detailed views of the abnormalities should be obtained (Fig. V-8a,b). Fetal radiography is most useful in the examination for a fetal skeletal dysplasia. However, even

when a skeletal defect is not suspected, a routine radiographic examination permits detection of anomalies that are difficult to demonstrate by dissection; these include abnormal vertebrae or hypoplasia/aplasia of individual bones (Ornoy et al., 1988). To detect abnormal development a familiarity with a normal pattern of ossification is important (Figs. V-9–12).

Histologic Examination

Histologic examination is necessary in order to identify such microscopic changes as aspiration of infected amniotic fluids into the lungs and deviations from normal development. Samples of all the internal organs should be submitted for histologic examination.

Examination of the Placenta

The placenta of conceptuses (9–18 developmental weeks) consists of an umbilical cord, extraembryonic membranes, a chorionic plate, and villi; each component should be carefully examined in every spontaneous abortion. Essential points in placental examination are placental weight (Appendix II, Table II-6), evaluation of both fetal and maternal placental surface, placental shape, site of insertion and length of the umbilical cord, the number of cord vessels, and the appearance of the placental membranes (see Chapter X). A histologic evaluation of membranes, the cord, and the chorionic villi near the fetal and the maternal surface should also be routinely made.

It should be remembered that, in all cases of fetal intrauterine death and prolonged retention, the placenta contains viable cells that can be used to initiate cell cultures for both metabolic disease diagnosis and cytogenetic studies, as well as for DNA studies.

Fig. V-6. An opened skull in preparation for brain fixation.

Fig. V-7. Set-up for photographic documentation.

Fig. V-8. (a) A preparation of a 17-week fetus with trisomy 21, for radiographic examination; A–P position, (b) Lateral view.

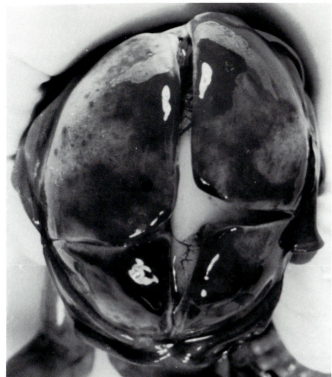

V-6

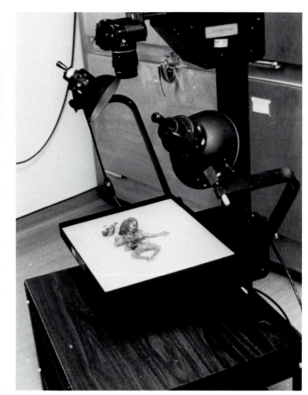

V-7

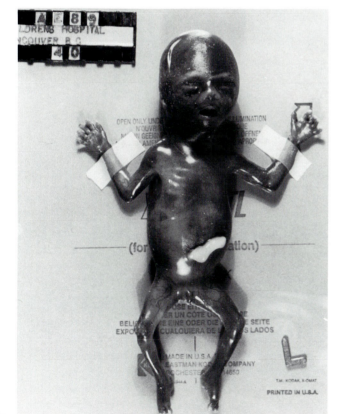

V-8a

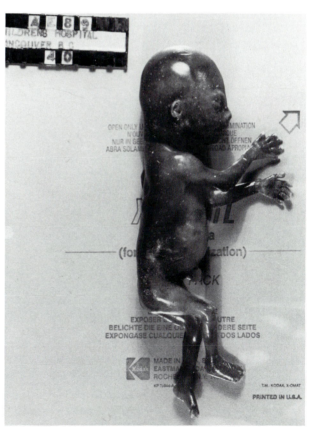

V-8b

Fig. V-9. Radiogram of a 12-week fetus (magnified); (a) A–P and (b) lateral position. The skull shows a well-ossified membranous calvarium. Mandibular ossification is incomplete in the midline, but the orbits are well developed. Spine: ossification of vertebral arches from the cervical to the lumbar region; primarily ossified vertebral bodies, thoracic and lumbar vertebrae, with a faint ossification beginning in the upper sacrum and lower cervical region. Chest: all 12 ribs ossified; well-defined clavicles appear at an angle. Hips: ilia with identifiable acetabular regions. Extremities: All long bones ossified; (not seen) all the short hand bones and all the short feet bones of the feet, except for the proximal and middle phalanges, show evidence of ossification.

Fig. V-10. Radiogram of a 14-fetus (actual size); (a) A–P and (b) lateral position. Skull: well-formed maxilla and mandible with tooth buds. Spine: definite ossification of cervical bodies above C_3 and below S_2. Chest: ribs further approximate vertebral arches but have not reached the sternum; clavicles and scapulae normally modeled. Hips: unchanged ilium, ischium slightly ossified. Extremities: Slight cupping of long bones persists; ossification of hands and feet continues; middle phalanges (hand) remain slightly smaller than the other phalanges.

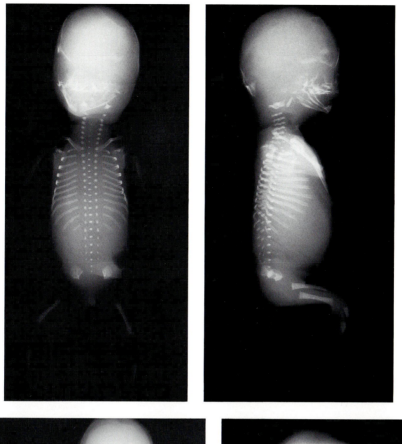

V-9a   *V-9b*

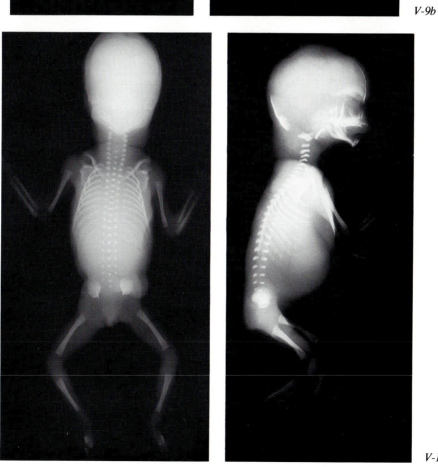

V-10a   *V-10b*

Fig. V-11. Radiogram of a 16-week fetus (reduced size); (a) A–P and (b) lateral position. Skull and face unchanged. Spine: vertebral bodies slightly larger. Chest: Eleven well-formed ribs extend anteriorly to the sternum, posteriorly to the vertebral arches. Clavicles and scapulae almost resemble those seen at term. Hips: Pelvis shows ossification of ischium. Extremities: ossification of all metacarpals, metatarsals, and phalanges (hands and feet).

Fig. V-12. Radiogram of a 18-week fetus (reduced size); (a) A–P and (b) lateral position. There is further growth in the length and width of all the bones; progressive ossification of ischium is the most noticeable change, compared to week 16.

C.
an

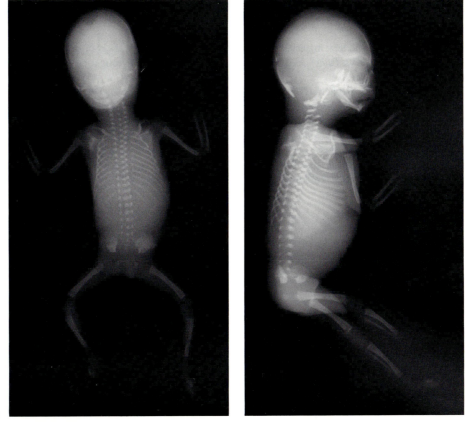

V-11a   *V-11b*

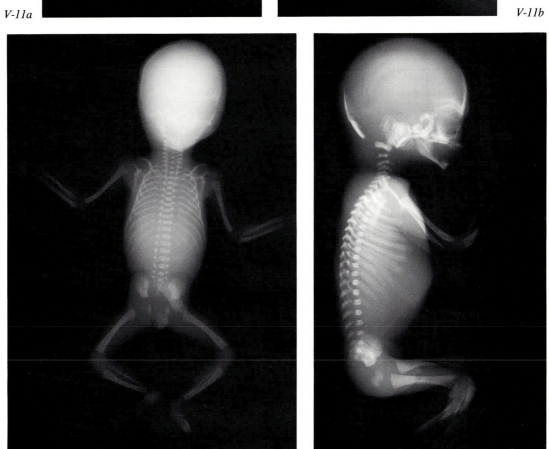

V-12a   *V-12b*

An intact sac containing a well-developed body stalk (5 mm in length) and either no embryonic tissue or a 2- to 3-mm nubbin of tissue attached to the free end of the stalk usually represents a conceptus in the GD_3 or GD_4 category, in which the abnormal embryo has become separated. On careful inspection, a necrotic area sealed with fibrin can be identified in the wall of such a chorionic sac, and occasionally a GD_3 or GD_4 embryo can be found outside the seemingly intact chorionic sac.

Fig. VI-1. Empty intact sac (GD_1); A, amniotic sac filled with fluid; C, opened chorionic sac. Note the absence of the embryo and yolk sac.

Fig. VI-2. A nodular embryo, 2 mm in length (GD_2); A/C, abnormal fusion of the amnion and chorion.

Fig. VI-3. A cylindrical embryo (GD_3); arrows, cephalic end with eye pigment.

Fig. VI-4. A stunted embryo (GD_4) with small head, dysplastic face, small head, absent cervical flexure, and delayed development of limb buds for CR length of 11 mm; Arrow, eye; F, fusion of chest and face; UL, upper limb.

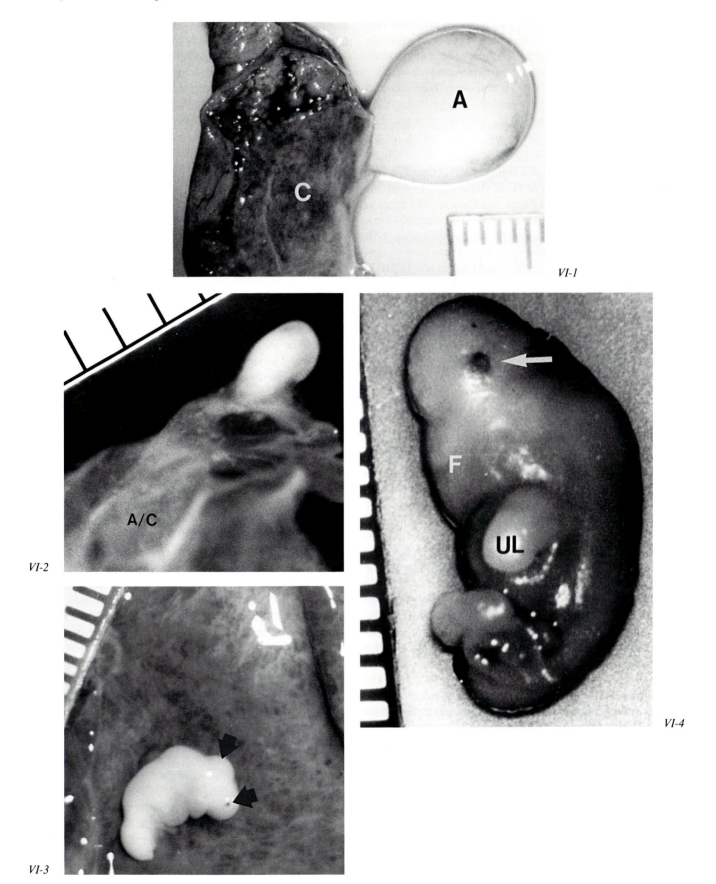

VI-1

VI-2

VI-3

VI-4

are more frequent and more severe, we will discuss these two defects separately.

Anencephaly Without Rachischisis

The anencephalic newborn has a unique appearance. The vault of the skull is missing and the brain tissue has degenerated into a spongy mass. Most of the bones at the base of the skull are abnormal. A typical head and facies include low-set ears with overfolded helices, proptosis, and large cheeks, nose, mouth, and tongue. The palate is often highly arched with deep grooves on both sides of the raphe. Other defects may involve a short neck, vertebral abnormalities, a shortened thorax, a large thymus, pulmonary hypoplasia, and such deformations of the limbs as clubfeet (talipes).

Most fetuses with anencephaly seen by a pathologist are from pregnancies that were terminated at 15 to 20 weeks. The anencephalic fetus resembles the newborn, except for the shape of the face, which typically has a triangular appearance. The palate is frequently arched. There is considerable variation in the size of the cranial defect. The pituitary fossa is usually flattened; and the optic nerves are usually small or absent.

The internal organs show variable defects (see Table VI-1). Hypoplasia of the adrenal cortex is a constant finding from 16 weeks of development. It is due to hypoplasia of the fetal zone caused by the absence of the hypothalamus and the consequent abnormal regulatory function of the pituitary gland.

Major additional malformations have been reported in all surveys of anencephalic fetuses and newborn. David and Nixon (1976), in a study of autopsy records of 158 newborn anencephalics without rachischisis found that 26% had additional abnormalities. Seller and Kalousek (1986) found additional major abnormalities in 19% of 52 anencephalic fetuses; in our group of 29 anencephalic fetuses, 38% had major additional abnormalities. These studies were combined and the data are summarized in Table VI-1.

Facial clefting and renal defects are most common. Renal defects consist of hydronephrosis, polycystic kidney, unilateral and bilateral agenesis, and unilateral hypoplasia. Skeletal defects include club hands and abnormal thumbs. Esophageal atresia and gut malrotation are among gastrointestinal defects. Heart defects vary from simple septal defects to complex transpositions. Hypospadias and a hypoplastic penis are among the genital defects.

TABLE VI.1. Major additional defects in 239 cases of anencephaly without rachischisis.

Defect	Percent
Cleft lip/palate	10.4
Renal defects	10.4
Skeletal Defects	4.6
Gastrointestinal defects	4.1
Heart defects	3.3
Genital defects	2.5
Omphalocele	1.6
Diaphragmatic hernia	0.8

Fig. VI-5. A posterior view of an embryo with anencephaly. The arrow indicates the hypervascular edge of the defect. Note the low-set, protruding ears.

Fig. VI-6. A spontaneously aborted, 8½-week-fetus with anencephaly; remnants of brain tissue and the leptomeninges (arrow).

Fig. VI-7. The separated head of a damaged, degenerated, 8½-week fetus with anencephaly; hypervascular area along the defect (arrows).

Fig. VI-8. A 15-week anencephalic, male fetus induced as a result of a prenatal diagnosis of anencephaly. Note the triangular face.

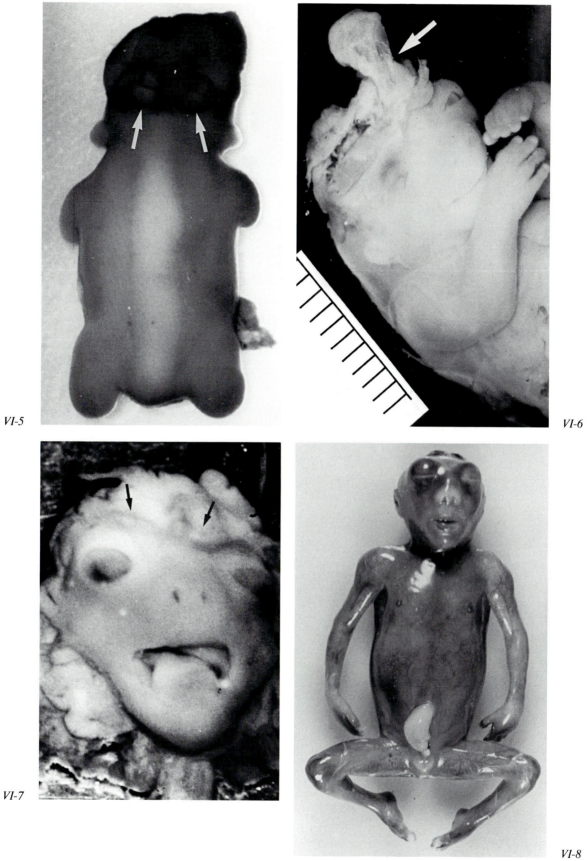

VI-5

VI-6

VI-7

VI-8

Fig. VI-9. A 16-week anencephalic fetus with meracrania.

Fig. VI-10. A 19-week anencephalic fetus with holacrania.

Fig. VI-11. A 16-week anencephalic male fetus with an unusual anterior extent of the lesion, resulting in anopthalmia.

Fig. VI-12. A 16-week anencephalic male fetus with cleft lip and palate.

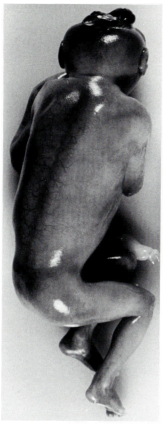

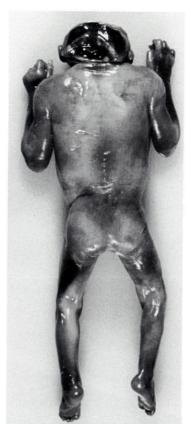

VI-9

VI-10

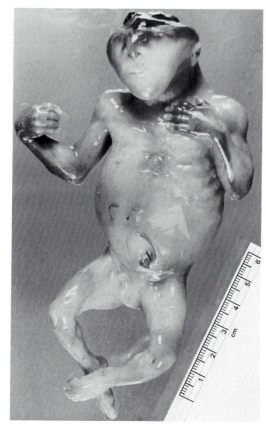

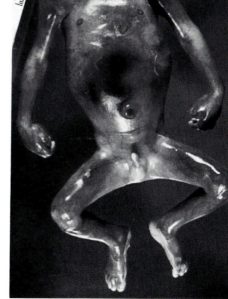

VI-11

VI-12

Anencephaly with Rachischisis

Estimates of the frequency at which anencephaly is accompanied by spinal rachischisis vary from 17 to 50% (David and Nixon, 1976). In this condition, not only does the anterior neural tube fail to close but also some or all of the body neural tube remains open. The size of the defect ranges from localization to the cervical area to the whole length of the neural tube. As with anencephaly alone, there is always adrenal hypoplasia. Vertebral defects, pulmonary hypoplasia, and clubfeet are more common in anencephaly with spinal rachischisis than in anencephaly alone. Usually the neck and thorax are shortened due to vertebral defects, and there may be scoliosis, which reduces the volume of the thorax and the abdomen. It has been suggested that shortening and deformation of the spine, due to abnormal development of the mesoderm surrounding the neural tube, predispose the embryo to more frequent major abnormalities such as renal defects, a dia-phragmatic hernia, omphalocele and congenital heart defects (Seller and Kalousek, 1986). In the largest series, which included 136 cases of anencephaly with spinal rachischisis (David and Nixon, 1976), renal defects were present in 17%, cleft lip and/or palate in 10%, gastrointestinal defects in 9%, omphalocele in 5%, diaphragm abnormalities in 5%, cardiovascular abnormalities in 4%, and spleen abnormalities in 2%.

There are approximately 20 cases in the literature in which anencephaly with spinal rachischisis is accompanied by cyclopia, proboscis, microphthalmia, a single nostril, and other features of holoprosencephaly (Lemire et al., 1981; Wolter et al., 1968). Since the facial features of the usual anencephalic fetus do not resemble holoprosencephalic facial features, this type of anencephaly probably has a different origin, which includes abnormal prechordal mesenchyme. Since so few cases have been described, the recurrence risk of this type of anencephaly is not known.

Fig. VI-13. A 15-week fetus with anencephaly and cervical rachischisis (arrow).

Fig. VI-14. A 16-week fetus with anencephaly and complete rachischisis.

Fig. VI-15. (a) A 17-week fetus with anencephaly, rachischisis, and multiple other developmental defects, including omphalocele, diaphragmatic hernia, and clubfeet. (b) Posterior view of the same fetus showing the extent of the spinal defect (arrows).

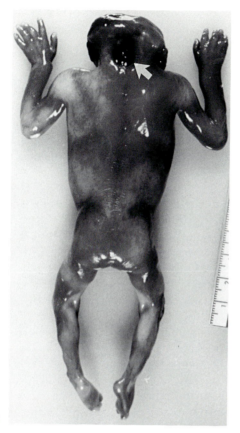

VI-13

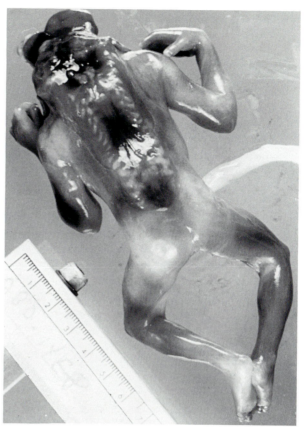

VI-14

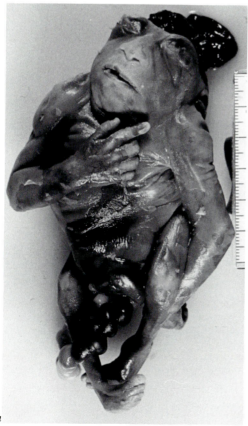

VI-15a

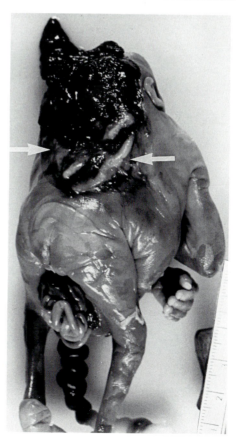

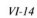

VI-15b

Myelocele

A defect due to the failure of the spinal neural tube to close, in which the neural tissue is exposed at the surface, is called a *myelocele*, or *rachischisis*. If the neural tissue is enclosed in a sac covered with arachnoid and dura, it is called a *myelomeningocele* or a *meningomyelocele*. If the sac contains only arachnoid and dura, it is called a *meningocele*. The most usual locations are lumbar or lumbosacral, but these lesions can occur anywhere along the spinal canal. About 50% of all CNS defects are myeloceles. The term *spina bifida* can be used for any of the above-described spinal defects and should therefore be avoided because it is not specific.

In embryos, myelocele has been found in triploidy and trisomy 16 (McFadden and Kalousek, 1989). In older conceptuses, myelocele or meningomyelocele have been associated with trisomy 13 and trisomy 18.

Myelocele is either due to a failure of closure of the spinal neural tube from the cervical to the midlumbar region or to abnormal canalization below the midlumbar region. A much more rare cause of lumbosacral myelocele is overgrowth of the neural plate tissue; this was first described by Patten (1952, 1953). This abnormality was observed and studied in detail by Kallen (1962) and Swinyard et al. (1973). It is frequently observed in the caudal region of embryos with chromosome defects (McFadden and Kalousek, 1989). It can appear as an overgrowth with surrounding pigmentation or a flat, placque-like protrusion in the caudal region. All 12 embryonic cases of neural overgrowth that have been cytogenetically analyzed were abnormal. Eight cases were triploid, and four were trisomy 13.

Myeloceles vary in location and size. They are most common in the lower thoracic, lumbar, and sacral regions. The neural canal can be open or covered by a thin membrane, or the neural tissue may be split longitudinally (Laurence, 1987). If the lesion is high up, the spinal cord caudal to the lesion is usually abnormal. There may also be cord abnormalities above the lesion; these include hydromyelia, diastematomyelia, diplomyelia, or syringomyelia.

From 10 to 20% of infants with myelocele have additional major defects (Khoury et al., 1982; Hall et al., 1988). There are more defects when the myelocele is above T_{11} (Toriello and Higgins, 1985; Seller and Kalousek, 1986; Hall et al., 1988) than when it is below T_{11}, where canalization defect is also involved. In live-born infants, Toriello and Higgins (1985) noted cleft lip and/or palate, unilateral renal agenesis, rib fusion, ventricular septal defect (VSD), an accessory spleen, and pelvic bone ossification defect in lesions at or above T_{11}, and rib fusion, aortic coarctation, renal agenesis, a short esophagus, a duplicated ureter, and an imperforate anus with lesions below T_{11}. Seller and Kalousek (1986) found that 90% of the upper spinal defect fetuses had associated abnormalities such as cleft lip and/or palate, congenital heart disease, and omphalocele. Of fetuses with the midspine defects, 30% had associated abnormalities such as an accessory spleen, a horseshoe kidney, Meckel's diverticulum, and malrotation of the gut. None of the cases with lower spine defects had any associated abnormalities.

Fig. VI-16. A 41-day embryo with thoracic and lumbar dysraphism (arrow) in the gestational sac. There is evidence of mild upper and lower limb growth retardation relative to the CR length.

Fig. VI-17. A 40- to 41-day embryo showing marked growth retardation of both the upper and lower limbs, facial dysplasia, and a large open defect (arrow) in the caudal portion of the neural tube. The karyotype was 69, XXY.

Fig. VI-18. A close-up view of an embryonic neural tube defect in the caudal region. Note the overgrowth of the neural folds and the complete failure of their closure (arrow); LL, lower limb buds; UL, upper limb buds.

Fig. VI-19. A midthoracic open neural tube defect (arrows) in an embryo (Stage 22) with a normal male karyotype.

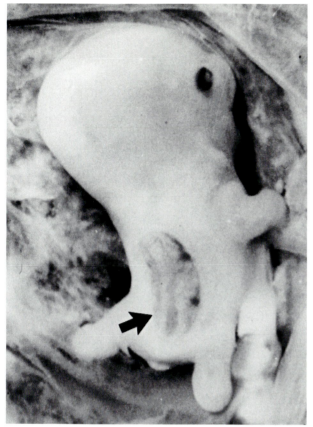

VI-16

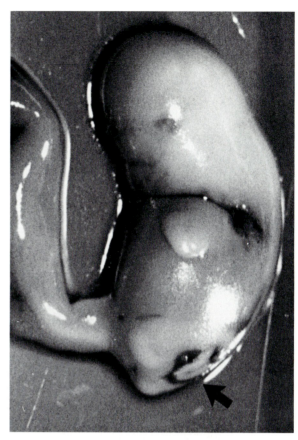

VI-17

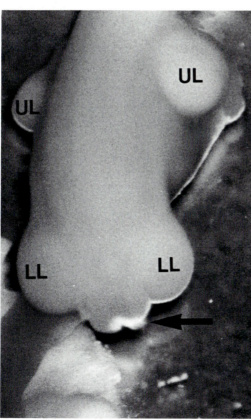

VI-18

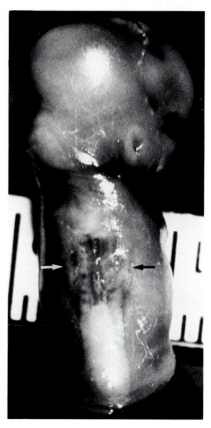

VI-19

Fig. VI-20. A 14-week male fetus with thoracolumbar myelocele and hydromyelia, arrow.

Fig. VI-21. An 18-week male fetus with a lumbosacral myelocele.

Fig. VI-22. A 19-week fetus with a lumbosacral meningocele associated with diplomyelia.

Fig. VI-23. A 20-week female fetus with lumbar myelocele and an intact sac.

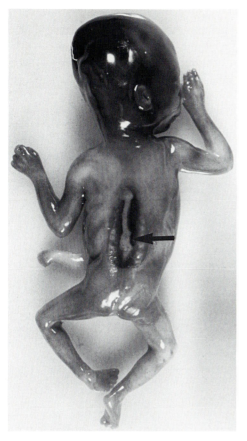

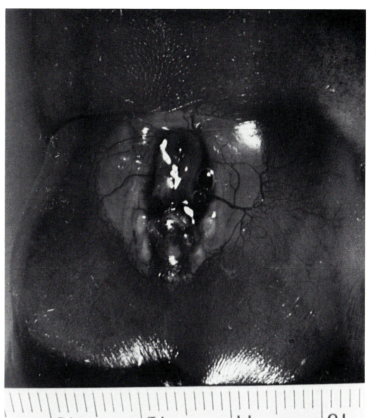

VI-20

VI-21

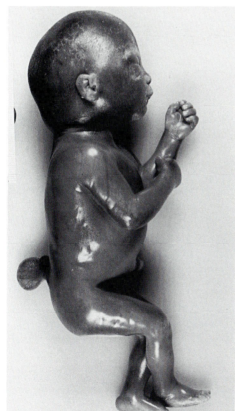

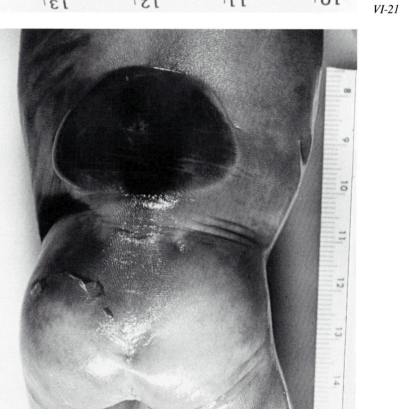

VI-22

VI-23

Iniencephaly

In this condition, the head is extremely retroflexed and the neck is absent. The face skin is continuous with the chest skin, and the posterior scalp is directly connected to the skin of the back. There may be a large encephalocele protruding from the open foramen magnum. There is often cleavage of the occipital region of the skull, and the occipital bone is found with the cervical vertebrae. The cervical vertebrae are always abnormal (abnormalities of shape and fusion), and the other vertebrae are often also abnormal. The skin of the neck and back is usually hirsute.

Iniencephaly is associated with additional malformations in 84% of the cases observed. Central nervous system abnormalities include anencephaly, hydrocephaly, and myelocele. There may be face abnormalities such as cyclopia, an absent mandible, and a cleft lip and palate. Renal malformations, for example, a horseshoe, ectopic, or polycystic kidney, are common. Cardiovascular and gastrointestinal malformations are also frequent, as is a diaphragmatic hernia (David and Nixon, 1976; Nishimura and Okamato, 1977).

Iniencephaly is a rare condition, but it is more common in geographic areas in which the anencephaly rate is high (Warkany, 1971). Like anencephaly, it is more common in females. A karyotypic abnormality was reported in one iniencephalic fetus; it was triploid (Byrne and Warburton, 1986).

Anencephaly may be associated with spinal retroflexion, and some investigators consider iniencephaly to be a variant of anencephaly. Others point out that many iniencephalics do not have anencephaly and that the neural tissue is covered with skin. Moreover, the incidence of associated abnormalities in anencephaly and iniencephaly is different (Warkany, 1971; Nishimura and Okamato, 1977).

Fig. VI-24. Lateral view of an embryo with iniencephaly. Note the absence of the neck and the direct attachment of the chin to the chest wall. The abdominal wall is damaged.

Fig. VI-25. A 12-week fetus with iniencephaly. Note the anencephaly with rachischisis; arrows point to eyes and nose.

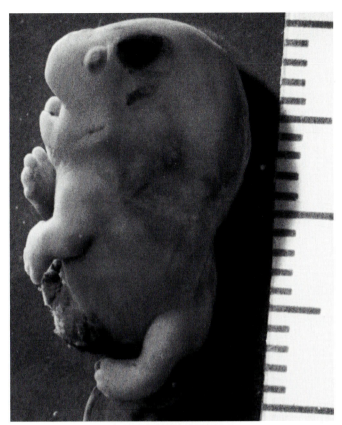

VI-24

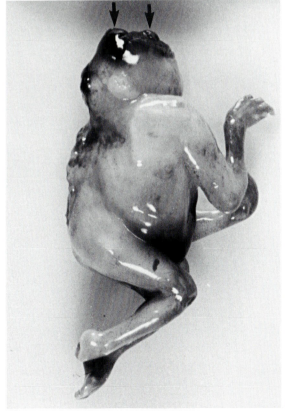

VI-25

Holoprosencephalic Disorders

This group of malformations consist of a combination of defects of the prosencephalon derivatives and of the midface (Demyer, 1977). Brain abnormalities range from relatively minor defects, consisting of absent olfactory bulbs, olfactory tracts, and trigones with an abnormal olfactory cortex, to a severe reduction in the growth of the prosencephalon, resulting in a small brain with a single ventricle and no cerebral hemispheres, corpus callosum, or septum pellucidum. There are all degrees of abnormality between these two extremes. The facial defects include various degrees of eye approximation and an absent or abnormal nose. Malformations of the upper lip can also occur. There may be a complete lack of separation of the eyes (cyclopia), with or without a proboscis, and an absent nose, or there may be extreme hypotelorism with or without a proboscis and absent nose (ethmocephaly). In cebocephaly, the hypotelorism is less severe and the nose is present but it has only one nostril.

The incidence of holoprosencephaly in newborns is between 0.02 and 0.006% (Chervenak et al., 1985). In embryos, it is higher, around 0.4% (Matsunaga and Shiota, 1977); thus, most holoprosencephalic conceptuses are eliminated before birth.

All the abnormal brain structures found in the holoprosencephalic spectrum are the result of abnormal growth and differentiation of the walls of the prosencephalon. The median face is derived from the mesenchyme ventral to the prosencephalon. There is evidence from animal studies that this prechordal mesenchyme induces the development of the anterior brain and there is an intimate relationship between midface development and the development of the optic and olfactory bulbs and the growth of the cerebral hemispheres. Abnormalities in development of this region have been described as the *holoprosencephaly sequence* (Jones, 1988).

This is an etiologically heterogeneous group (Cohen, 1982, 1989). Many different chromosome abnormalities have been reported, the most common being trisomy 13 or 13 q⁻. Other chromosome abnormalities observed in holoprosencephaly include duplications and deletions of chromosome 18, trisomy 21, and triploidy (Munke et al., 1988). Table VI-2 lists some of the more common genetic syndromes associated with holoprosencephaly (Cohen, 1982).

TABLE VI.2. Genetic conditions with holoprosencephaly (adapted from Cohen, 1982).

Syndrome	Features
Dominant inheritance	
Autosomal dominant holoprosencephaly	Variable expression
Autosomal recessive	
Autosomal–recessive holoprosencephaly	Typical facial dysmorphism
Agnathia–holoprosencephaly	Variable expression
Holoprosencephaly–endocrine dysgenesis	Facial clefts, genital hypoplasia, endocrine dysgenesis
Fryns syndrome	Diaphragm defects, absent/hypoplastic fingernails and distal phalanges, cloudy cornea
Meckel–Gruber syndrome	May have holoprosencephaly or encephalocele, polydactyly, polycystic kidneys

Fig. VI-26. A diagram of different types of facial defects in holoprosencephaly.

Fig. VI-27. A 15-week female fetus with holoprosencephaly and proboscis (arrow), partial cyclopia (a fused orbit and two eyes), and a small mouth. Note the edema of the scalp and neck.

Fig. VI-28. A 17½-week fetus with trisomy 13. Note the hypotelorism and the single nostril.

Fig. VI-29. A degenerated 18-week fetus with trisomy 13. Note the hypotelorism, absent nose, and median cleft lip.

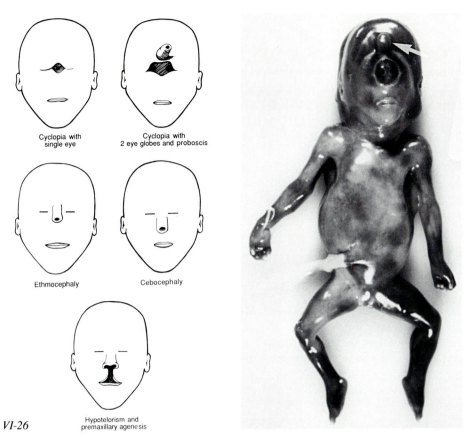

Cyclopia with
single eye

Cyclopia with
2 eye globes and proboscis

Ethmocephaly

Cebocephaly

Hypotelorism and
premaxillary agenesis

VI-26

VI-27

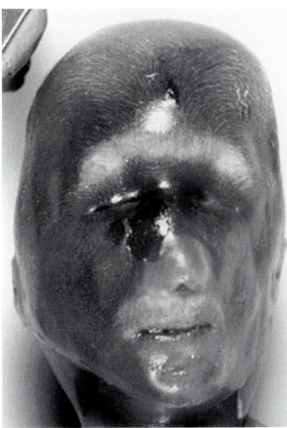

VI-28

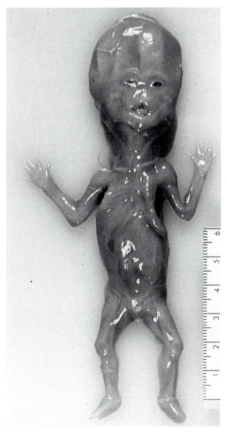

VI-29

Cephalocele

In cephalocele, the intracranial contents protrude through a bony defect of the skull. When brain tissue is in the herniated sac, it is called an *encephalocele*. The term *cranial meningocele* is used when only meninges are herniated. The incidence is 0.3 to 0.6 in 1000 live births (Lorber, 1966). In the newborn, the defect usually occurs in the occipital area. In the embryo, the mesencephalic component of the occipital area is in the parietal area, and it is displaced as the cerebral hemispheres develop (Leong and Shaw, 1979). It seems likely that a variety of neural tube or mesenchyme abnormalities could cause this defect, but its etiology is not known at present.

Encephalocele occurs in many syndromes. Table VI-3, and occasionally in some chromosome abnormalities. It is associated with maternal rubella, hyperthermia, and diabetes.

We have found encephaloceles in chromosomally normal embryos and in embryos with triploidy, trisomy 14, trisomy 15, and 45,X. Within each group, locations can be frontal, parietal, or occipital. In some cases, the encephalocele was typical, in others it appeared as a solid bulge of tissue. In the latter instance, there is some generalized degeneration of the embryo and, presumably, these atypical defects were originally typical encephaloceles.

In occipital encephalocele, the bony defect may include the foramen magnum and the posterior arch of the atlas. The brainstem is often abnormal and the spinal cord may show developmental defects. Occipital encephalocele is common in iniencephaly and in the Meckel-Gruber syndrome.

Encephalocele may also occur in the parietal and anterior regions (Warkany et al., 1981). Parietal encephaloceles are usually midline, and the associated abnormalities may be an absent corpus callosum, a Dandy–Walker defect, or other brain malformations. An anterior encephalocele may be visible or externally invisible, and the amount of brain tissue present within the sac varies greatly. With all types of encephaloceles, there may be an associated microcrania or a hydrocephaly.

Other associated defects may be meningomyelocele, cleft palate, or congenital heart disease.

TABLE VI.3. Syndromes with encephaloceles (from Cohen M, Lemire R (1982)).

Amniotic band syndrome
  Multiple encephaloceles (predominantly anterior), constriction and amputation of digits or limbs, polydactyly, syndactyly, facial disruptions, cleft lip/palate
Walker–Warburg syndrome (HARD- or Chemke syndrome or cerebrooculodysplasia)
  Occipital encephaloceles, hydrocephaly, cerebellar dysgenesis, agyria, retinal dysplasia, cataracts, congenital muscular dystrophy
Cryptophthalmos syndrome (Fraser syndrome)
  Occipital encephalocele, one or both eyes covered by skin, syndactyly of hands and/or feet
Dyssegmental dwarfism
  Occipital encephalocele, narrow chest, reduced joint mobility, abnormal vertebrae, short bent limbs
Frontonasal dysplasia
  Frontal encephalocele, hypertelorism, anterior cranium bifidum occultum, widely set nostrils
Knoblock syndrome
  Occipital encephalocele, vitroretinal degeneration, meningocele
Meckel-Gruber syndrome
  Occipital encephalocele, polydactyly, polycystic kidneys, holoprosencephaly, microphthalmia, hepatic bile duct proliferation
Von Voss syndrome
  Occipital encephalocele, phocomelia, urogenital anomalies, absent corpus callosum
Warfarin syndrome
  Occipital encephalocele, limb shortening, hydrocephaly, nasal hypoplasia
Associations
  Absent corpus callosum, cleft lip/palate, craniostenosis, Dandy–Walker malformation, Arnold–Chiari malformation, ectrodactyly, hemifacial microsomia, iniencephaly, Klippel–Feil syndrome, meningomyelocele

Cohen and Lemire (1982) reviewed the syndromes and associations with cephaloceles (Table VI-3). An encephalocele produced by an amniotic band is shown in Figure VI-120.

Fig. VI-30. A trisomy 14, 39-day embryo, with a large parietooccipital encephalocele (arrow). Other anomalies include a small head and delayed development of the upper and lower limb buds and tail. Two large cysts are attached to the umbilical cord.

Fig. VI-31. An embryo (Stage 20) with parietal and occipital encephaloceles (arrows); the karyotype is normal.

Fig. VI-32. An embryo (Stage 21) with a large occipital encephalocele (arrow) in an intact amniotic sac.

Fig. VI-33. A 14-week fetus with a large occipital encephalocele in an intact sac.

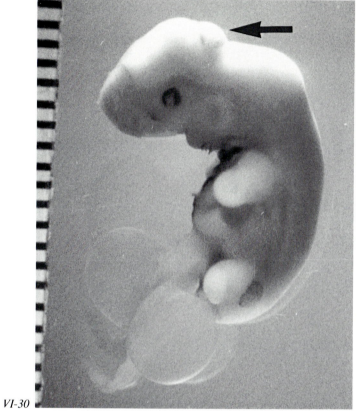

VI-30

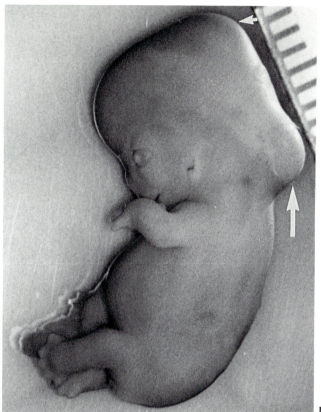

VI-31

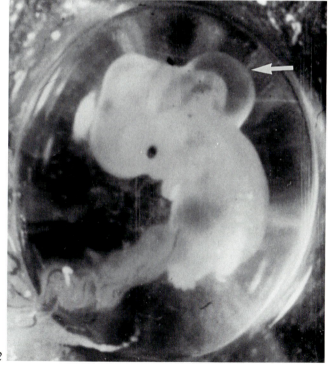

VI-32

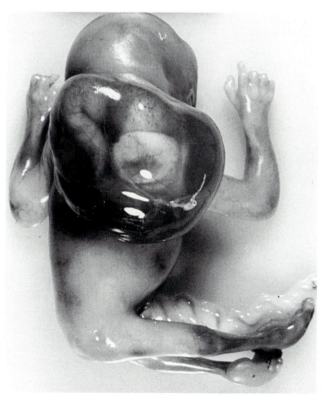

VI-33

Fig. VI-34. A 15-week fetus with a parietal encephalocele.

Fig. VI-35. A 16½-week fetus with an occipital encephalocele in a damaged sac.

Fig. VI-36. An 18-week male fetus with Meckel-Gruber syndrome. Note the large occipital encephalocele, polydactyly and protruding abdomen.

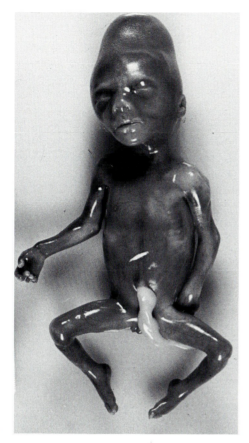

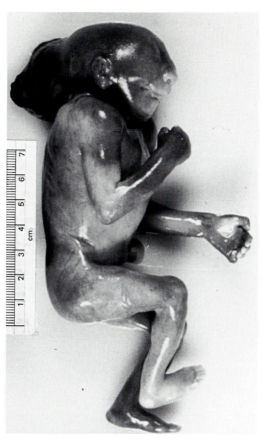

VI-34

VI-35

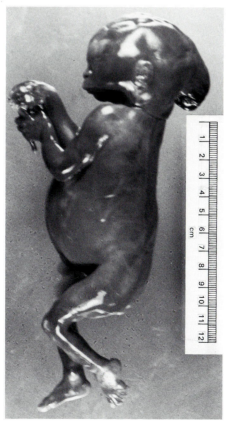

VI-36

Hydrocephalus

Hydrocephalus is an increase in the amount of intraventricular cerebrospinal fluid (CSF). It is usually due to an obstruction. The incidence varies from 0.3 to 2.5 per 1000 live births.

Theoretically, the increase in the amount of CSF may be due to overproduction of CSF, defective absorption of CSF, or obstruction of the CSF pathway (Laurence, 1987), but in previable period the vast majority of cases are due to obstruction. Ex vacuo hydrocephalus, due to a loss of brain tissue, has not been described in previable fetuses.

There are many possible causes of obstruction. The aqueduct of Sylvius may be narrowed or malformed. There may be malformations of the hindbrain such as the Arnold–Chiari malformation, in which the cerebellar vermis protrudes through the foramen magnum and the medulla is displaced past the foramen magnum to obstruct CSF flow. This malformation is commonly seen with myelocele, and has been detected as early as the tenth week of gestation. The Dandy–Walker malformation, another cause of hydrocephalus, consists of a hypoplastic or an absent cerebellar vermis and an enlarged fourth ventricle separating widely the cerebral hemispheres. The foramina of Magendie and Luschka are absent from the abnormal roof of the ventricle.

Hydrocephalus can develop early in the second trimester of pregnancy or it may not develop until after birth. It may be associated with a variety of infections, or mutant genes. An X-linked recessive aqueductal stenosis occurs in about 2% of cases in which there are no other abnormalities. Hydrocephalus may also be inherited as a dominant or a multifactorial condition (deLange, 1977). It may also be part of such syndromes as achondroplasia, osteogenesis imperfecta, the Hurler syndrome, or, rarely, tuberous sclerosis.

Fig. VI-37. (a) A 17-week fetus with hydrocephalus and no other developmental defects; normal male karyotype. (b) Lateral view of the same fetus. (c) Brain section of the same fetus, showing enlargement of the ventricles and reduced amount of brain tissue.

Fig. VI-38. (a) A 15-week male fetus with hydrocephalus and multiple developmental defects consisting of pulmonary hypoplasia, malrotation of the bowel, absent vertebral bodies C_{1-2}, and clubfeet. The karyotype is normal. (b) Lateral view of the same fetus.

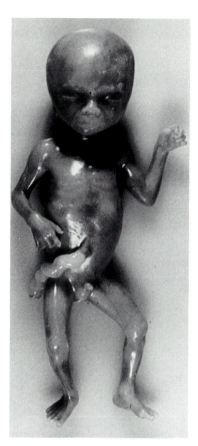
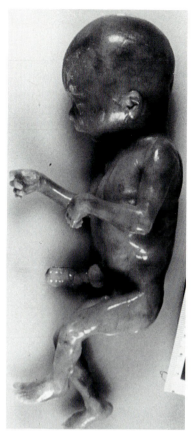
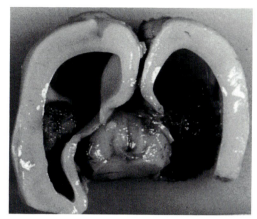

VI-37a

VI-37b

VI-37c

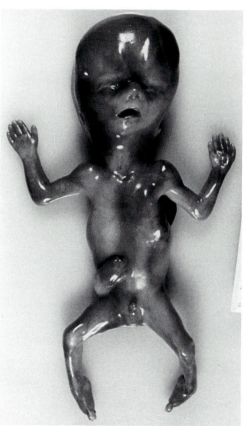
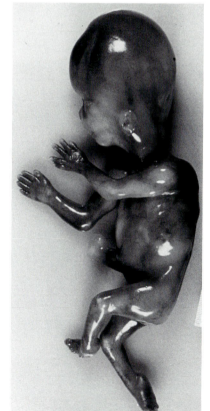

VI-38a

VI-38b

Microcephaly

Microcephaly has been defined in some studies as a head circumference smaller than 2 standard deviations (SD) below the mean; in other studies, 3 SD is used. It varies in degree from mild to severe. In newborns, isolated microcephaly is present in about 1 in 6200 to 1 in 40,000 live births (Warkany et al., 1951). In embryos with chromosome abnormalities such as trisomy 9, 13, 14, 18, 22 finding, microcephaly is common. Microcephaly is rare in spontaneously aborted, chromosomally normal fetuses. Ultrasound intrauterine diagnosis of fetal microcephaly and termination of microcephalic fetuses are feasible. Some of the causes of microcephaly are listed in Table VI-4.

TABLE VI.4. Classification of microcephaly

Microcephaly without associated malformations
  Genetic: Primary microcephaly, Paine syndrome, Alpers disease
  Environmental: Radiation exposure, malnutrition, trauma, hypoxia
Microcephaly with associated malformations
  Chromosomal abnormalities: Trisomy 9, 13, 18, 21, 22, abnormalities of chromosomes 1–5, 7–15 and 22
  Gene defects: Many syndromes
  Environmental: Infections; prenatal exposure to alcohol, drugs, or chemicals; maternal phenylketonuria

From Ross J, Frias J: Microcephaly, in Vinken P, and Bruyn G (eds): Congenital Malformations of the Brain and Skull, Handbook of Clinical Neurology: Amsterdam, Elsevier, North Holland Publishing Co. Vol. 30 p. 507–524, 1977.

Fig. VI-39. A Stage 18 embryo with microcephaly. Note the lack of a frontal prominence; C, Cystic cord.

Fig. VI-40. A 15½-week triploid fetus with severe microcephaly.

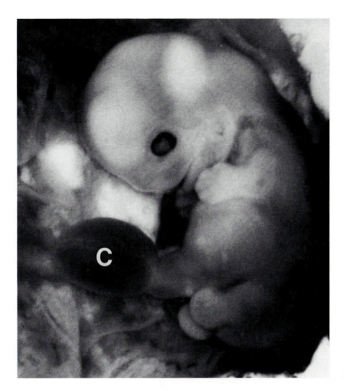

VI-39

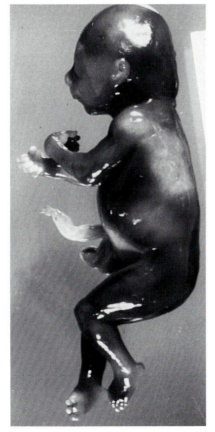

VI-40

FACIAL CLEFTS

Introduction

Definition and Types

The term *facial clefts* refers to a wide spectrum of facial cleft-ing. These clefts are usually at the site of fusion of the fron-tonasal, maxillary, and mandibular prominences and produce lateral or median cleft lips with or without a cleft palate. Irregular facial clefts may be produced by amniotic bands.

Incidence

In the newborn, facial clefting is a common congenital mal-formation. Lateral cleft lip and/or palate is found in one of 700 liveborns. Approximately 50% of these have both cleft lip and/or palate, 25% have cleft lip only, and 25% have cleft palate only. Median cleft lip accounts for only 0.2 to 0.7% of cases of cleft lip. In aborted embryos and fetuses, facial clefts are rare unless there is a chromosome abnormality.

Embryology and Pathogenesis

Cleft Lip

Lateral Cleft Lip

During the fifth week of gestation, the nasal pits are bounded by the medial and lateral nasal swellings. The maxillary swellings develop lateral to these two swellings and eventu-ally fuse with both of them. The medial nasal swelling will form the philtrum and part of the upper lip. Fusion of the medial nasal swellings with the maxillary swellings occurs during the sixth and seventh week (Stage 18), and failure of fusion will result in cleft lip. The cleft may be limited to the lip or may extend, in various degrees, to the nose. It may be unilateral or bilateral. The diagnosis of cleft lip in embryos can be made only upon completion of the seventh week of development.

Median Cleft Lip

The medial nasal swellings merge during the sixth and seventh week, and failure of fusion will result in median cleft lip. It is interesting to note that median cleft lip can be associated with hypotelorism in the holoprosencephaly spec-

trum or hypertelorism in the median cleft face sequence. The latter is a sequence that results in severe ocular hyper-telorism, a frontal bone deficit, a notched or bifid nose, and a median cleft lip and palate (Smith 1982). It is possible that in the hypotelorism of holoprosencephaly, there is a defi-ciency of mesodermal tissue; in the hypertelorism of the median cleft face sequence, there may be a slower approxima-tion of the bilateral nasal swellings.

Cleft Palate

The palate arises from a small midline anterior part that is formed from the medial nasal prominence (primary palate) and the secondary palate that arises from the deeper part of the maxillary swellings. In the seventh and eighth week of development, the palatine shelves, which have formed from the maxillary swellings, move above the tongue and fuse with each other and the primary palate. Fusion is complete by about the 8th to the 10th week of development. Interference with growth or movement of the palatine shelves could pro-duce cleft palate. Failure of fusion of the medial and maxil-lary swellings (cleft lip) may disturb secondary palatal closure, and cleft palate is often associated with cleft lip. Isolated cleft palate, especially in a partial form, can be diag-nosed only upon completion of 10 weeks of development.

Etiology

Facial clefts are etiologically a very heterogenous group. Lateral cleft lip and/or cleft palate may occur as isolated abnormalities or as part of a syndrome. Isolated cleft lip with or without cleft palate is a different entity from cleft palate alone and has a different recurrence risk. Referral to the clini-cal genetics service of the family after diagnosis of cleft lip or palate in a chromosomally normal conceptus for a complete evaluation is important, since inheritance may be dominant, X-linked, or multifactorial.

Cleft lip and palate are found in 10 to 50% of cases of trisomy 18 in the newborn. In our trisomy 18 group of fetuses, 12% had cleft lip and/or cleft palate. In trisomy 13, over 50% of newborns have facial clefts (Smith, 1982); in our group of trisomy 13 fetuses, 55% had facial clefts. Other chromosome abnormalities may be associated with facial clefts as well.

The etiology of median cleft lip associated with the holo-prosencephaly syndrome is heterogeneous. At the present time, nothing is known about the etiology of the median cleft face sequence.

Irregular facial clefts or those occurring in atypical loca-tions are usually produced by amniotic bands; this is dis-cussed later in the chapter.

Pathology

In the embryo, cleft lip cannot be recognized until after seven weeks, since fusion does not occur until that time. If the embryo is examined shortly after Stage 18 and autolysis is severe, the newly fused tissue may degenerate and an artifactual cleft may appear. Thus, cleft lip cannot be diagnosed in a severely autolyzed embryo. This is not the case in fetuses in which fusion is well established.

Morphologically, lateral, median, and irregular facial clefts are readily distinguished. Lateral clefts may be unilateral or bilateral. The clefting caused by amniotic bands is usually bizarre and may involve the oral, nasal, and orbital cavities. It is always asymmetric. In the presence of cleft lip, careful external and internal examinations and chromosomal analysis are indicated.

Cleft palate can only be diagnosed after embryonic period, since the hard palate starts closing after the eighth week of development. The posterior soft palate closes after the 9th

week, and the uvula remains bifid until the 10th week of development. The degree of clefting can vary from a notch to a full-thickness cleft.

Since cleft palate can occur as an isolated defect, it is always important to examine the palate.

Associated Abnormalities

Some of the syndromes in which cleft lip and/or palate may be seen are presented in Tables VI-5 and VI-6.

TABLE VI.6. Syndromes in which cleft palate alone is common (adapted from Cohen, 1983).

Syndrome	Features
Autosomal Recessive	
Camptomelic	Bowing of femora and tibiae
de la Chapelle	Micromelia, short curved radius and ulna
Christian	Craniosynostosis, arythrogryposis
Cleft palate/brachial plexus neuritis	Facial asymmetry, deep-set eyes, hypotelorism, recurrent brachial plexus neuritis
Cleft palate/connective tissue dysplasia	(? X-Linked), cervical fusions, dislocated radial heads, clinodactyly
Cleft palate/stapes fixation	Skeletal anomalies, stapes fixation
Diastrophic dysplasia	Contractures, hitchhiker's thumb, deformed ear
Dubowitz	Microcephaly, blepharophimosis
Lowry–Miller	Persistent truncus arteriosus, abnormal right pulmonary artery
Majewski	Short narrow thorax, polydactyly of hands and feet
Micrognathic dwarfism	Micromelia, cleft vertebrae
Multiple pterygia	Multiple pterygia
Palant	Microcephaly, bulbous nasal tip, toe clinodactyly
Rudiger	Hand flexion contracture, small fingers and fingernails
Wallace	Short limbs, hydrocephalus
Weaver–Williams	Midface hypoplasia, bone hypoplasia, delayed osseous maturation
Automal Dominant	
Abruzzo–Erickson	(? X-Linked dominant) Coloboma, large ears, hypospadia
Apert	Craniosynostosis, midface deficiency, hand and foot syndactyly
Cerebroco-stomandibular	Robin anomaly, upper thoracic deformity
Cleft palate/lateral synechiae	Lateral synechiae

TABLE VI.5. Syndromes in which cleft lip/palate are common (adapted from Cohen, 1983).

Syndrome	Features
Autosomal Recessive	
Appelt	Tetraphocomelia, enlarged penis/clitoris
Bixler	Microtia, ectopic kidneys, heart defect
Bowen–Armstrong	Toe syndactyly, ankyloblepharon filiforme, hyperpigmented areas
Crane–Heise	Low-set ears, absent cervical vertebrae and clavicle, finger and toe syndactyly
Juberg–Hayward	Microcephaly, hypoplastic distally placed thumbs, short radii
Meckel-Gruber	Polydactyly, polycystic kidney, encephalocele
Michel	Blepharophimosis, ocular chamber defect, short fifth fingers
Varadi	Polydactyly, arrhinencephaly, heart defect
Autosomal Dominant	
Clefting/ankyloblepharon	Ankyloblepharon filiforme
Ectrodactyly–ectodermal dysplasia	Hand and foot ectrodactyly
Martin	Microcephaly, hypotelorism, absent premaxilla, spinal anomalies
Popliteal pterygium	Popliteal pterygia, hypoplastic digits
Rapp-Hodgkin	Dystrophic nails, thin wiry hair
van der Woude	Lip pits
Unknown Genesis	
Clefting/ectropion	Ectropion lower eyelids, limb reduction defects

continued

TABLE VI.6. (*Continued*).

Syndrome	Features
Autosomal Dominant	
Ectrodactyly cleft palate	Ectrodactyly; syndactyly, hands and feet
Gordon	Camptodactyly, clubfoot
Kniest	Dwarfism, kyphoscoliosis, tibial bowing
Wildevanck	Cervical fusion
X-Linked	
Orofacialdigital	Bifid tongue, dystopia canthorum, brachydactyly
Otopalatodigital I	Frontal prominence, short terminal phalanges and nails, curved toes
Otopalatodigital II	Microstomia, flexed overlapping fingers, hypertelorism
Persistent left superior vena cava	Persistent left superior vena cava, ASD (atrial septal defect), clubfoot
Unknown Genesis	
Femoral hypoplasia—unusual facies	Short nose, short/absent femurs and fibulas
Klippel–Feil	Fusion of cervical vertebrae
de Lange	Microbrachycephaly, confluent eyebrows, limb anomalies

Fig. VI-41. Diagram showing fusion of palatine shelves (8th to 10th week of development).

Fig. VI-42. Embryo (Stage 22) with trisomy 13. Note the large median cleft lip.

Fig. VI-43. Embryo (Stage 22) with triploidy. Note the unusual median cleft lip with normal growth of the lateral prominences at the margins of the cleft. Eye coloboma is also present.

Fig. VI-44. Degenerated embryo, Stage 19, with bilateral cleft lip. Note the degeneration of the corners of the mouth, but no evidence of any artifact in the cleft area; T, protruding tongue.

Fig. VI-45. A 9-week fetus with a median cleft lip.

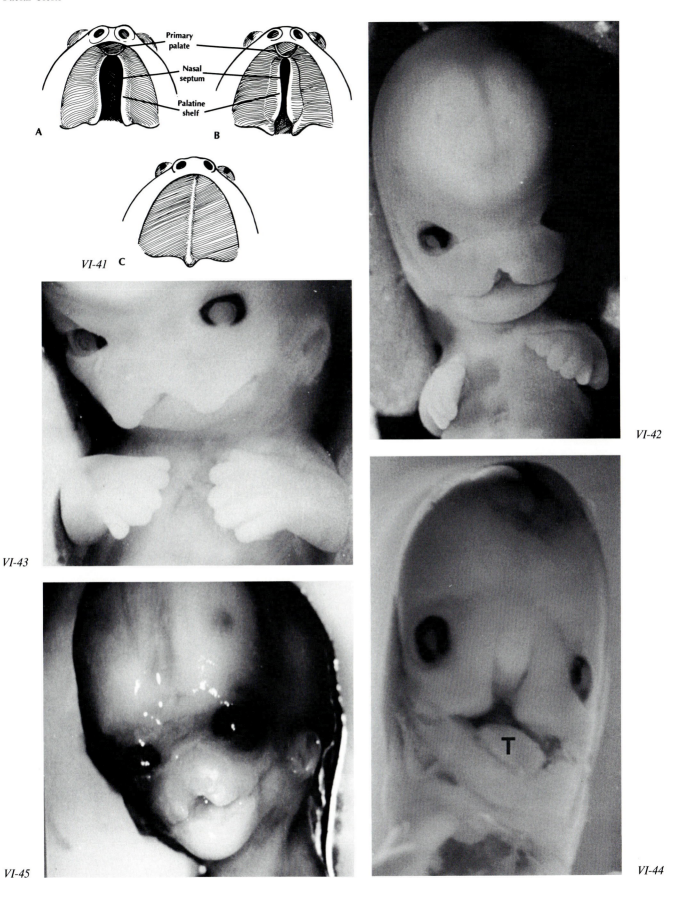

VI-41

Primary palate

Nasal septum

Palatine shelf

A

B

C

VI-42

VI-43

VI-45

T

VI-44

Fig. VI-46. A degenerated 10-week fetus with a bilateral cleft lip and palate. The right eye is partially reopened due to degeneration. A slit in a lower lip is an artifact.

Fig. VI-47. A fresh, 13-week male fetus with a bilateral cleft lip and palate.

Fig. VI-48. A fresh, 20-week fetus with Fryn's syndrome. Note the large right cleft lip and palate.

Fig. VI-49. A fresh, 20-week fetus with a unilateral left cleft lip.

Fig. VI-50. A 14-week female with asymmetric facial clefting due to amniotic bands.

Fig. VI-51. (a) An embryo (Stage 22) with a neural tube anterior palate defect showing a well-formed upper lip and normally positioned posterior palatal shelves prior to their fusion; T, tongue; arrow, deficiency of premaxilla. (b) mouth of a 16-week fetus opened with forceps to show clefting of both the hard and soft palates. There is no defect of the upper lip; N, nostrils; T, tongue.

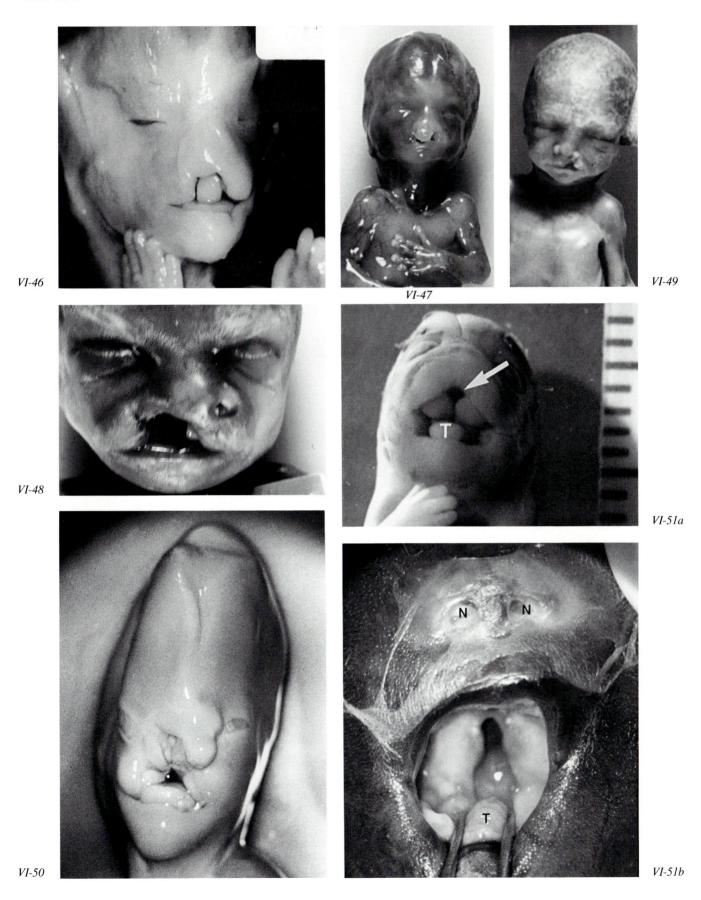

VI-46

VI-47

VI-49

VI-48

VI-51a

VI-50

VI-51b

Limb Abnormalities

Introduction

Limb abnormalities may be divided into bone abnormalities and contractures (arthrogryposis), which are due to neurologic or muscle disease. In the embryo, with the exception of syndactyly, polydactyly, and complete limb agenesis, very few limb abnormalities can be identified. Between 8 and 12 weeks of gestation, the lower limb development lags behind that of the upper limb. After 12 weeks, the lower and upper limbs are equally developed. Because of the availability of ultrasound to detect skeletal defects the pathologist can now see a wide variety of early fetal limb defects. Examination of a fetus with limb defects must include full-body X-rays and cartilage, bone, and connective tissue specimens for histologic and electron microscope studies.

Skeletal dysplasias have been classified by an international working group (Romero et al., 1988) and the existing classification is complicated. Skeletal dysplasias are divided into osteochondrodysplasias, dysostoses, idiopathic osteolyses, miscellaneous disorders with osseous involvement, chromosome aberrations, and primary metabolic abnormalities. In this section, we discuss only a few limb abnormalities such as limb contractures and sirenomelia. Osteochondrodysplasias (achondrogenesis and osteogenesis imperfecta), some dysostoses and hypophosphatasia are illustrated. The reader is referred to Spranger et al. (1974), Temtamy and McKusick (1978) for further information on skeletal dysplasias.

The dysostoses are divided into three different groups. One of them is dysostosis with a predominant involvement of extremities. Syndactyly, polydactyly and reduction deformity are included in this group. Polydactyly is one of the most common limb abnormalities in the embryo and fetus under 20 weeks and often occurs in trisomy 13. Polydactyly may be on the radial (preaxial) or the ulnar (postaxial) side. Preaxial polydactyly ranges from a bifurcation of the tip of the thumb to a duplicated thumb or index finger or both. On the postaxial side, the additional digit ranges from a skin tag on the fifth finger to an extra finger. Syndactyly often occurs with polydactyly. Some definitions used in describing reduction deformities are presented in Table VI-7.

TABLE VI.7. Some terms used in describing reduction deformity.

Acromelia	Distal shortening of a limb
Mesomelia	Shortening of middle segment of limb
Rhizomelia	Proximal shortening of limb
Hemimelia	Absence of a longitudinal segment
Amelia	Complete absence of a limb
Acheira	Absence of a hand
Apodia	Absence of a foot
Adactyly	Absent finger(s)

Limb Contractures

Limb Contractures Without Pterygia

Fixation of a joint is thought to be due to a failure of mobility in embryonic and/or fetal life. There are many possible causes of immobility, both extrinsic and intrinsic. Among the extrinsic causes are bicornuate uterus, tubal pregnancy, twinning, and oligohydramnios. Intrinsic causes are abnormalities of the brain, spinal cord, muscle, skin (e.g., ichthyosis), and connective tissue.

Animal experiments have shown that reduced fetal movement has other effects as well. Growth is usually retarded, the heart and lung are hypoplastic, the umbilical cord is short, and often there is polyhydramnios. This group of abnormalities is called the *fetal akinesia deformation sequence* (Moessinger, 1983). Reduced breathing movements lead to pulmonary hypoplasia, reduced swallowing may allow polyhydramnios, and decreased movement of the fetus can affect cord length.

Any factor that reduces fetal mobility will result in the fetal akinesia deformation sequence (FADS) in varying degrees, so one would expect it to be an element in many different syndromes. One of the first such syndromes was described by Pena and Shokeir (1974), and the FADS is sometimes designated the Pena–Shokeir phenotype. At present, many reports involve FADS (Hall, 1986), but the various syndromes have not yet been clearly delineated. When a fetus with limb contractures is studied, it is important to identify the cause of fetal immobility by a careful study of the brain, spinal cord, muscle, connective tissue, and placenta.

Fig. VI-52. (a) A 15-week female fetus with achondrogenesis (Type II). All the limbs are reduced in length and the thorax is small. (b) A radiogram of the same fetus showing absent ossification of most vertebrae, shortened long bones, and irregular, spurred metaphyses (84% actual size).

Fig. VI-53. (a) A 15-week female with osteogenesis imperfecta (Type IIA). The philtrum appears long; limbs are short and deformed. (b) A radiogram of the same fetus. Note the reduced ossification of the calvarium, short beaded ribs, and short broad limb bones with multiple fractures (89% actual size).

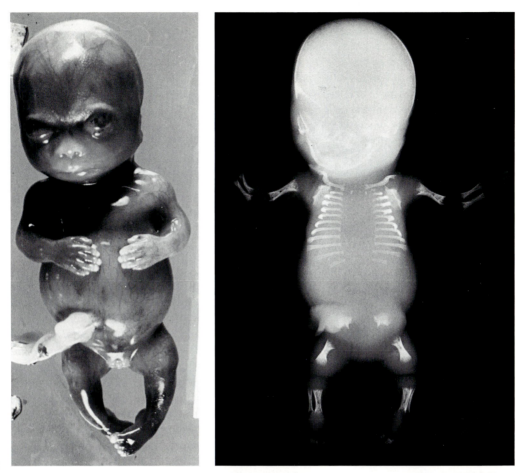

VI-52a   *VI-52b*

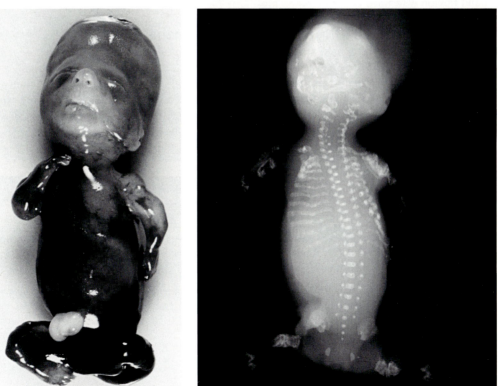

VI-53a   *VI-53b*

usually absent and the iliac bones are usually fused. The anus is imperforate and the kidneys, ureters, bladder, urethra, and external genitalia are absent.

The abnormality that produces this defect must occur in the first few weeks of development and has often been thought to be due to a wedge-shaped abnormality at the caudal end of the primitive streak. Kampmeier (1927) reviewed 79 cases of sirenomelia and described the blood vessel abnormalities that are part of the syndrome. There is only one "umbilical artery," which arises high in the aorta. After this vessel arises, the aorta and its branches continue as very slender vessels. The "umbilical artery" is probably one of the vitelline vessels that continues into the umbilical cord in the absence of a true umbilical vessel. Kampmeier suggested that the reduced blood supply may cause sirenomelia. However, the role of vascular malformations is not yet clear. Frequently, there are deformities in the anterior part of the body that cannot be explained by abnormal vitelline vessels. Furthermore, sirenomelia is over 100 times as common in monozygotic twins as in dizygotic twins or singletons (Smith et al., 1976), which suggests that a deficiency of caudal tissue may be an early abnormality.

Agenesis of the Lower Spine

This group of syndromes is characterized by varying degrees of developmental failure of the spinal cord and vertebrae. The sacral and coccygeal vertebrae and sometimes the lumbar vertebrae are abnormal or missing. The legs may be short and there may be abduction and flexion deformities at the hips and knees, which result in the frogleg position. There may also be renal agenesis, congenital heart deformities, gastrointestinal defects, cleft lip (palate), microcephaly, and spina bifida. In about 16%, the mothers of these infants were diabetic (Gellis and Feingold, 1968).

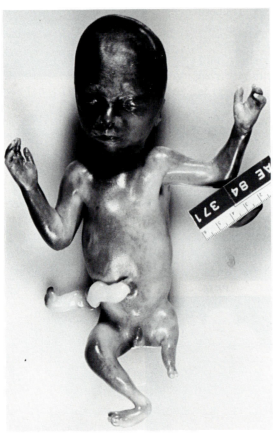
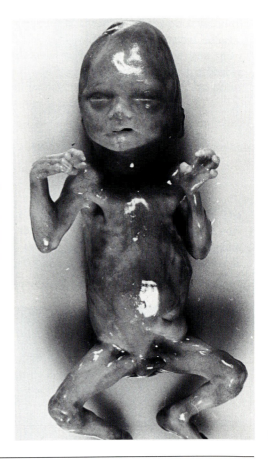

VI-59   *VI-6*

Fig. VI-59. A 20-week fetus with an absent left femur, tibia, and fibula; a hypoplastic right femur and an absent right fibula.

Fig. VI-60. A 17-week male fetus, with a normal chromosomal complement, showing contractures of the wrists and fingers.

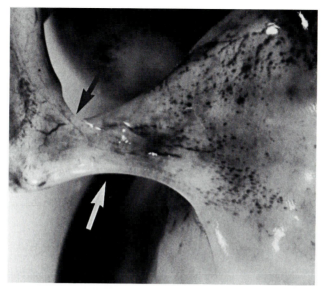

VI-62

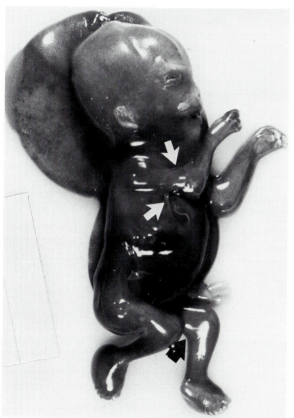

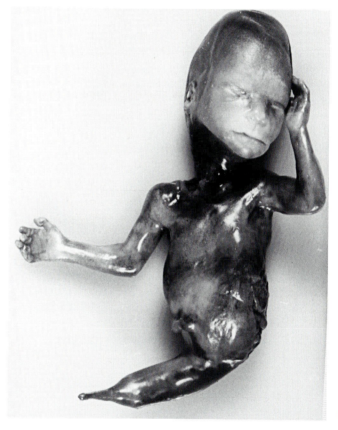

VI-61

VI-63

Fig. VI-61. A macerated 15½-week fetus, with the lethal multiple pterygium syndrome, demonstrating the classical phenotype with posterior cervical cystic hygroma and axillary, cubital, and popliteal pterygia (arrows). Note the muscle wasting in all the extremities.

Fig. VI-62. Axillary and cubital webs (arrows) in a 14½-week male with the lethal multiple pterygium syndrome.

Fig. VI-63. A 17-week male fetus, with sirenomelia. The fetus had anal atresia and absent external genitalia, kidneys, ureters, urinary bladder, urethra, and rectum.

Abdominal Wall Defects

Introduction

The two most common defects of the abdominal wall are omphalocele and gastroschisis. Of these, omphalocele is seen more frequently. The karyotype is usually normal in gastroschisis, whereas about 50% of prenatally diagnosed omphalocele cases have an abnormal karyotype.

Omphalocele

Definition

Omphalocele (exomphalos) is a herniation of the intestine and sometimes other abdominal organs through the intact umbilicus into the umbilical cord. The sac containing the abdominal contents is lined with peritoneum, which has fused with the amnion of the umbilical cord. The umbilical cord may be located either at the apex of the sac, in small omphaloceles, or it may arise from the inferior border of the sac, in larger omphaloceles.

Incidence

The incidence in liveborn infants is approximately 1 in 6500 births. About one half of newborn infants with omphalocele are stillborn. If these stillborns are included, the incidence is one in 3200 (McKeown et al., 1953). In spontaneous abortions, the omphalocele is usually associated with chromosome abnormalities, CNS defects, or the amnion rupture sequence. An isolated omphalocele in a chromosomally normal fetus is a rare finding among spontaneous abortuses.

Types

Dott (1932) divided omphaloceles into two types, small and large, which are morphologically different and probably arise in different ways. Small omphaloceles usually contain only intestine and the umbilical cord arises from the apex of the sac. The umbilical ring is enlarged but normally placed. In the large omphaloceles, the abdominal wall superior to the umbilicus is absent and the sac may contain liver and other abdominal organs in addition to the midgut. In the large omphaloceles, the umbilical cord arises from the inferior aspect of the sac. Most investigators have not differentiated between these two types. An exception is Aitken (1963), who found that small omphaloceles were three times as common as large ones in liveborn infants.

Embryology and Pathogenesis

It is probable that the two types of omphaloceles arise in different ways. In normal development, 6 weeks after fertilization, the midgut passes out of the abdominal cavity at the base of the umbilical cord and returns to the abdominal cavity in the 10th week. This physiological herniation of the midgut does not include any other organs. If the midgut fails to return, the result is a small omphalocele.

In contrast, larger omphaloceles are associated with an absence of tissue superior to the umbilical cord. In normal development, the two lateral folds grow ventrally and medially and eventually fuse in the midline. Any disturbance in lateral fold growth could produce a weakness above the umbilical cord and permit extrusion of the liver, the pancreas, and the other organs that are often seen in large omphaloceles.

Etiology

About 50% of fetuses with omphalocele diagnosed prenatally have an abnormal karyotype (Gilbert and Nicolaides, 1987; Mann et al., 1984). Trisomy 18 is common; triploidy, trisomy 13, trisomy 21, 45,X, and XXY have also been reported.

Mendelian inheritance is rare in omphalocele. Osuna and Lindham (1976) have described one family with dominant inheritance of omphalocele. A recessive form in which all the siblings died during the first year of life was reported by Czeizel and Vitez (1981), and an X-linked recessive may be the form of inheritance in the family described by Havalad et al. (1979).

In the amnion rupture sequence and limb body wall complex, omphalocele is a frequent finding; it is also common in the Beckwith-Wiedemann syndrome (Beckwith, 1969).

Fig. VI-64. An embryo (Stage 22), showing a physiological umbilical hernia.

Fig. VI-65. A 10-week fetus with a large segment of small bowel herniated into the umbilical cord. At this stage of development, the complete bowel should be in the abdomen.

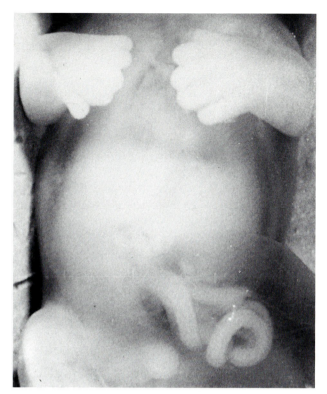

VI-64

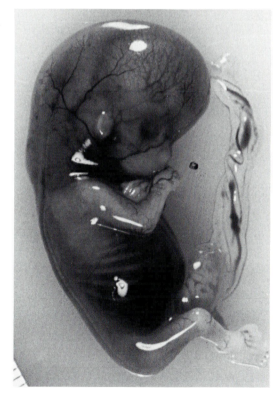

VI-65

Syndromes and Other Associated Malformations

Approximately 50% of infants with non-Mendelian omphaloceles have other abnormalities (Czeizel and Vitez, 1981; McKeown et al., 1953; Mann et al., 1984). Almost all affected infants have some degree of intestinal malrotation because the gut has not returned to the abdomen, and rotation could not be completed. Other gastrointestinal abnormalities, such as pyloric stenosis and atresias, have been reported, and cardiovascular malformations are frequent. Greenwood et al. (1974), in a study of 37 patients with omphalocele and a cardiac defect, noted that the most frequent lesion was the tetralogy of Fallot, followed in frequency by a secundum type of atrial septal defect. Genitourinary, skeletal, CNS, and diaphragmatic abnormalities are often described, as are cleft lip and palate (Czeizel and Vitez, 1981). A rarer combination of abnormalities consists of exstrophy of the colon and bladder, spine and genitourinary abnormalities (Carey et al., 1978).

Cantrell et al. (1958) described a syndrome of supraumbilical midline abdominal wall defects that also includes abnormalities of the sternum, diaphragm, pericardium, and heart. Omphalocele is a common finding in this pentalogy of Cantrell.

Pathology

Since some of the gut is extraabdominal until the 10th week of development, small omphaloceles cannot be diagnosed until this time. The external surface of the sac around the gut in the omphalocele consists of amnion only.

The small sacs contain loops of small intestine and occasionally stomach and/or a part of the liver. The large sacs may have the spleen, liver, pancreas, or kidney, in addition to small and large bowel loops. If the sac has ruptured in utero, secondary changes such as edema of the bowel wall can occur.

Fig. VI-66. A 17-week fetus with a small omphalocele that contains only a few loops of the small bowel.

Fig. VI-67. A 19-week male fetus with an omphalocele that contains the small bowel, the right colon and part of the liver, spleen, and stomach.

Fig. VI-68. A 17-week female fetus with an omphalocele that contains the small bowel and liver.

Fig. VI-69. A macerated 10½-week fetus with an amnion rupture sequence and a large omphalocele. Note the amniotic band entanglement of the left foot and both hands and the facial clefting. The omphalocele contains mainly liver.

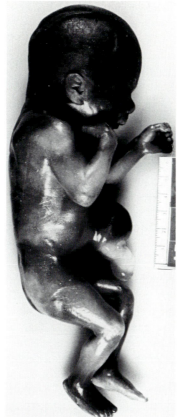

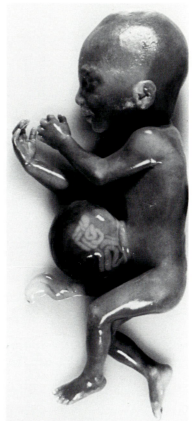

VI-66

VI-67

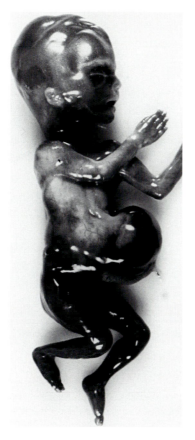

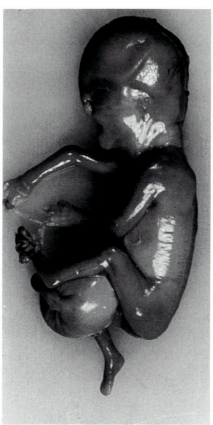

VI-68

VI-69

Gastroschisis

Definition

Gastroschisis is an abdominal wall defect that permits herniation of the abdominal organs. The defect is usually on the right side of the umbilicus and may extend into the bladder area. The umbilical cord is not involved in this defect, and there is no sac covering the exposed viscera.

Incidence

Gastroschisis occurs in about one in 12,000 live births (Baird and MacDonald, 1981).

Embryology and Pathogenesis

In normal development, at Stage 13 (28 days), the right and left umbilical veins drain the placenta, body stalk, and abdominal wall (deVries, 1980). The entire right umbilical vein, except for a remnant just below the vena cava, has atrophied by 33 days. The nutritive function of this vessel is taken over by the vitelline arteries. At first, two vitelline (omphalomesenteric) arteries (right and left) are present; the left one later atrophies and the right one becomes the superior mesenteric artery. DeVries suggests that either premature atrophy or abnormal persistence of the right umbilical vein could produce partial anoxia of the abdominal wall. If the right vitelline artery is disrupted (Hoyme et al., 1981), this would have the same effect on the abdominal wall; both these hypotheses would explain why gastroschisis usually occurs on the right side of the umbilicus. Vascular accidents of the omphalomesenteric artery would result in defects of other organs supplied by this vessel, that is, another result of blood vessel damage could be gastrointestinal atresia and stenosis.

Etiology

Gastroschisis is usually a sporadic defect that has not been associated with any chromosome abnormalities. However, there have been a few reports of sibling gastroschisis in families in which other family members occasionally had abdominal hernias (Salinas et al., 1979), which suggests a possible genetic etiology in such cases.

Pathology

Gastroschisis differs from omphalocele mainly in that the umbilical cord is not involved and that no sac or sac remnants are present. Sections of the adjacent abdominal wall should be taken to document muscle abnormalities. It is important for genetic counseling that gastroschisis be differentiated clearly from omphalocele because gastroschisis is usually sporadic whereas omphalocele is often part of a syndrome.

Gastroschisis in previable fetuses comes to the pathologist's attention after prenatal detection and pregnancy termination. Since this defect is not associated with chromosomal aberrations, it is usually not observed in spontaneous abortuses.

Associated Syndromes and Abnormalities

Such gastrointestinal defects as atresia and stenosis frequently accompany gastroschisis, and defects of other organ systems have been found in 24% of liveborn with gastroschisis (Baird and MacDonald, 1981). Mann et al. (1984), Hoyme et al. (1981), and Warkany (1971) have reported cases with heart, diaphragm, sternum, kidney, and CNS abnormalities.

Fig. VI-70. A diagram showing the abdominal wall blood supply. If the arterial supply or the venous drainage is disrupted, gastroschisis may result.

Fig. VI-71. A 15-week female fetus with gastroschisis and a normal chromosomal complement. Note the normal insertion of the cord and the abdominal wall defect on the right side; S, stomach; L, liver.

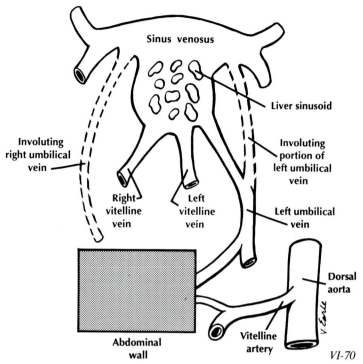

VI-70

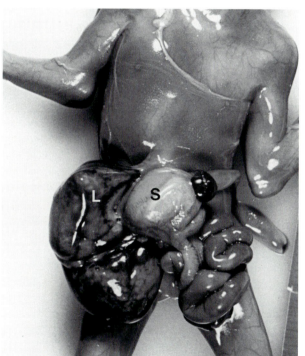

VI-71

DEFECTS OF THE DIAPHRAGM

Introduction

Two main types of abnormalities can give rise to diaphragmatic defects. One type consists of either *unilateral* or *bilateral agenesis*, or gaps of variable sizes in the posterolateral or retrosternal area. A gap in the posterolateral area is usually at the foramen of Bochdalek; a retrosternal gap at the foramen of Morgagni. In the other type of defect, the diaphragm is complete, but weak, due to a reduced number of muscle fibers. This type is called *eventration of the diaphragm.*

Incidence

Diaphragmatic defects occur in 0.03 to 0.05% of births (Romero et al., 1988). Of these, 85 to 90% are the Bochdalek hernias, which are usually on the left side. About 1 to 2% are Morgagni hernias, which are usually on the right side. About 5% are eventrations of the diaphragm. Unilateral and bilateral agenesis of the diaphragm are rare.

Etiology

Chromosome Abnormalities

There are a few reports of diaphragmatic hernia with trisomies 13, 18, or 21 (David and Illingworth, 1976; Puri and Gorman, 1984), ring 4 (Hansen et al., 1984), 45,X (Bonham Carter et al., 1962), and tetraploidy 21 (Benacerraf and Adzick, 1987). Banacerraf and Adzick (1987) found chromosomal abnormalities in 21% of 19 patients with a diaphragmatic defect.

Genetic Factors

More than 60 familial cases of diaphragmatic defects or agenesis have been reported (Norio et al., 1984). Most data are compatible with multifactorial inheritance, but a few cases may be autosomal recessive. Diaphragmatic defects may occur as part of a syndrome, for example, Beckwith-Wiedemann (Thorburn et al., 1970) or Frýns syndrome (Fryns et al., 1979). Occasionally, such defects may be present in the Ivemark or Goltz–Gorlin syndromes (Wolff, 1980).

Eventration of the diaphragm may be the result of muscle diseases, for example, an X-linked centronuclear myopathy or myotonic dystrophy (Moerman, 1987) and has been described in siblings (Schubert-Staudacher and Jauch, 1984).

Embryology and Pathogenesis

In the sixth week of development, the abdominal and thoracic cavities are partially separated. The septum transversum occupies the anterior part of the developing diaphragm. The central part is composed of the esophageal mesentery, and lateral to this mesentery are the pleuroperitoneal folds. The space between the pleuroperitoneal folds and the esophageal mesentery is called the pericardioperitoneal canal. At this stage, the abdominal and thoracic cavities communicate through these canals. The left canal is more extensive than the right canal (Wells, 1954). With further growth of the embryo, these spaces are obliterated, and the primitive diaphragm is complete by the eighth week of development (Hamilton et al., 1978). Further development of the diaphragm occurs by contribution from the body wall. Some of the myoblasts that form the diaphragm muscles migrate from the body wall, others are formed in situ (Wells, 1954).

If fusion of the pleuroperitoneal membrane with the esophageal mesentery and the septum transversum is not complete, a gap that can allow abdominal contents into the thorax is present. This defect is usually unilateral and on the left. It is called a hernia through the foramen of Bochdalek, although Wells (1954) pointed out that this is a misnomer, since Bochdalek actually described lumbocostal triangles, not the gap that is seen if failure of fusion occurs.

Another site of hernia is in the intersternocostal triangle. This is located between the muscle fibers that come from the xiphoid cartilage (pars sternalis) and neighboring fibers (pars costales). The gap is called the *foramen of Morgagni*, and the liver and other abdominal organs may herniate through it.

In diaphragmatic agenesis, one half or both halves may be absent.

Pathology

The diaphragm completes its development during the embryonic period, so a diaphragmatic gap seen in the fetal period is a diaphragmatic defect. In Bochdalek hernias, abdominal organs such as the stomach, spleen, and intestine can be seen in the thoracic cavity. Since these hernias usually occur on the left, the heart and lungs are compressed toward the right. This affects the growth of the lungs and their vasculature, to produce pulmonary hypoplasia. The number of conducting airways is reduced, as is the number of blood vessels. Malrotation of the bowel also occurs.

The Morgagni hernia is usually smaller than the Bochdalek hernias, and it usually occurs on the right side. The liver and, occasionally, other abdominal organs may have herniated into the thorax.

In diaphragmatic agenesis, the liver, stomach, and most of other abdominal organs may be in the thorax. Apart from displacement and malrotation of abdominal organs, the main pathology in diaphragmatic agenesis is again pulmonary hypoplasia.

Associated Abnormalities

Pentalogy of Cantrell (1958) describes the association of abdominal wall defect and the defects of sternum, diaphragm,

pericardium and heart. The diaphragmatic defect in this syndrome is always ventral (Toyama, 1972).

About 50% of infants with diaphragmatic abnormalities have associated defects (David and Illingworth, 1976). In a study of 143 cases, 28% had nervous system defects; 20% gastrointestinal defects; 15%, genitourinary defects; 13%, cardiovascular defects; 12%, skeletal defects; and 13%, other defects. The nervous system defects most commonly associated with diaphragmatic defects are myelocele, with or without anencephaly, and hydrocephalus (David and Nixon, 1976). Greenwood et al. (1976) found that 23% of infants with diaphragmatic defects had variable cardiovascular abnormalities with no one type being predominant.

Most iniencephalic infants have diaphragmatic defects. The distortion of body form that is so obvious in iniencephalic fetuses suggests that one cause of the failure to obliterate the pleuroperitoneal canals may be their distortion due to the abnormal body form.

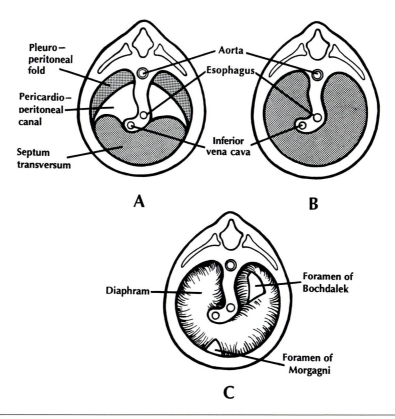

Fig. VI-72. A diagram of the development of diaphragm (A,B) and positioning of foramina Bochdalek and Morgagni (C).

In normal development, the atrial cavity is first divided into two parts by the growth of the septum primum from the superior wall of the atrium and by the upward growth of a septum from the endocardial cushions. The space between them is the ostium primum, which is obliterated when the septa fuse. Fenestrated openings form in the septum primum and join together to form the ostium secundum. Another septum, the septum secundum, grows next to the septum primum in the seventh week. It grows downwards towards the endocardial cushions to partially overlap the ostium secundum, leaving a smaller opening called the *foramen ovale*.

Pathology

There are three types of ASD. The most common are ostium secundum defects; the sinus venosus defect is the most rare. *Ostium secundum defects* are due to the failure of the septum secundum to occlude the foramen secundum. The *atrioventricular region defect* is usually a part of an atrioventricular septal defect. The *sinus venosus defect* is either located high in the interatrial septum near the entrance of the superior vena cava or, more rarely, near the entrance of the inferior vena cava.

Ventricular Septal Defects

Definition and Embryology

A *ventricular septal defect* (VSD) is the result of an incomplete separation of the right and left ventricle.

The cardiac ventricle is divided into right and left sections by the growth of a septum from the floor of the ventricles, the two truncoconal ridges, and the posterior atrioventricular (AV) endocardial cushion.

Pathology

Ventricular septal defects, existing in isolation or as part of other lesions, are the most common type of heart malformation. The commonest type, classified as *perimembranous*, predominantly involve the area of the central fibrous body. The second most common type is the *muscular septal* defect. Muscular defects occur in all parts of the septum, and may be multiple. *Infundibular* defects, the least common, lie directly under the pulmonary and aortic orifices that form part of the edge of the defect. Multiple defects combining all three types may occur.

Atrioventricular Septal Defects

Definition and Embryology

Atrioventricular septal defects (AVSD) include a spectrum of cardiac malformations involving, to different extents, the atrial and ventricular septa and the atrioventricular valves.

In normal development, the mesenchymal thickenings and endocardial cushions on the walls of the AV canal fuse. This divides the canal into right and left orifices. The mesenchyme tissue around each orifice differentiates into the bicuspid (mitral) valve on the left and the tricuspid valve on the right.

Pathology

Developmental defects of the AV canal involve both the atrial and the ventricular septa. There are three types. In the least severe form, there is an ostium primum defect but the tricuspid and mitral orifices are separate. Usually there is a cleft between the anterior and posterior leaflets of the mitral valve. A second type is an incomplete, persistent, common AV

Fig. VI-76. A perimembranous interventricular septal defect (arrow) in a 19½-week female fetus.

Fig. VI-77. A muscular ventricular septal defect (arrow) in a macerated 11-week female fetus, with trisomy 18.

Fig. VI-78. Two ventricular septal defects—large muscular (M) and perimembraneous (arrow)—in a macerated 13-week female fetus with multiple developmental anomalies.

Fig. VI-79. A complete, large AV canal defect in a 17-week male fetus with trisomy 21. Note the tissue bridge between the anterior and posterior valvular leaflets (arrow).

Fig. VI-80. A complete AV canal defect in an 18-week female fetus with trisomy 21. There is also a large atrial septal defect, secundum type (arrow).

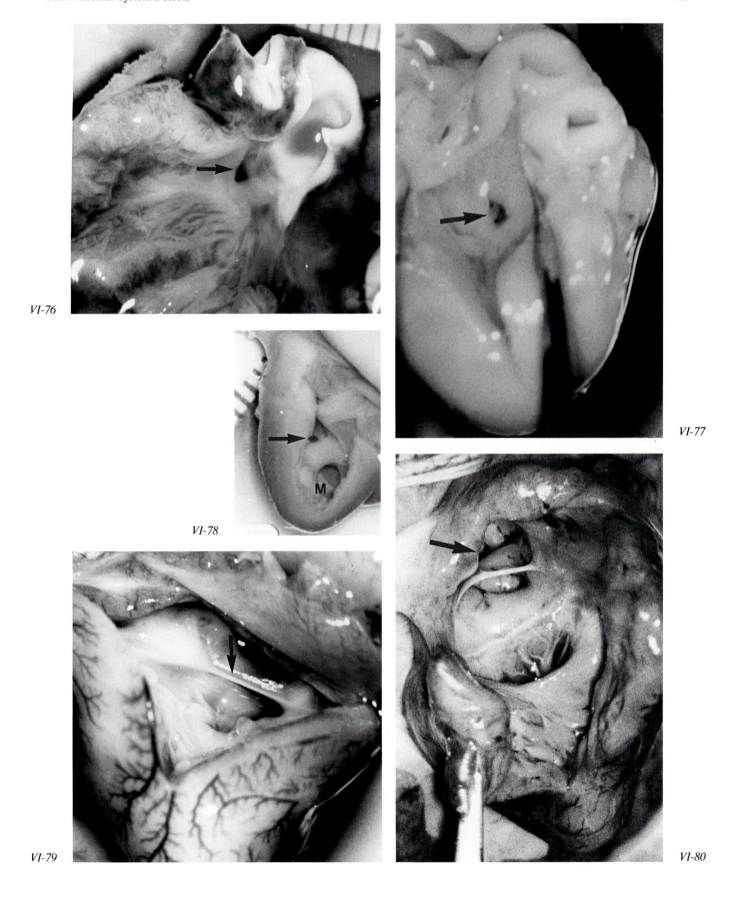

VI-76

VI-77

VI-78

VI-79

VI-80

canal, which includes the defects of the first type plus a bridging of the valve tissue from the anterior to the posterior position of the valves. The third type is a complete, persistent, common AV canal in which there is only one AV orifice with one valve and five leaflets. There is an associated defect in the atrial and ventricular septum.

The AVSD are often seen together with other cardiac defects, such as aortic coarctation, tetralogy of Fallot, pulmonary stenosis or atresia, and the asplenia and polysplenia syndromes. In the trisomy 21 syndrome, the second type of the AVSD described above is most commonly found.

Abnormal Basic Connections of the Heart

Abnormalities of the basic connections of the heart represent the minority of heart malformations. In principle, they can be defined as abnormalities in the basic structure and interconnectedness of the atria, ventricles, and great arteries (Van Praagh, 1972). There are three ways in which the two atrial chambers with their appendages can be misarranged: mirror image, an isomerism of right type, and an isomerism of the left type. Abnormal atrioventricular connections can be classified as concordant, discordant, and ambiguous. Abnormal

ventriculoarterial connections are common and are frequently asociated with other intracardiac lesions such as VSD, mitral valve atresia, and atrioventricular septal defect (Anderson and Allan, 1989).

Coarctation of the Aorta; Interruption of the Aortic Arch

Coarctation of the aorta is defined as a narrowing of the lumen. This can occur in any location along the course of the vessel but is most commonly seen in the distal aortic arch in the previable fetus. This usually takes the form of a uniform, tubular narrowing proximal to the ductus arteriosus. It must be differentiated from a physiologic narrowing of the isthmus of the aorta, which represents two thirds of the diameter of the ascending aorta. Other cardiac malformations are often associated with a coarctation of the aorta, which predisposes to a reduced aortic flow, as in a hypoplastic left ventricle, VSD, and a bicuspid aortic valve. In 45,X fetuses, tubular hypoplasia is almost always present.

The extreme form of coarctation of the aorta is the interruption of a segment of the aortic arch (Ho et al., 1983).

Fig. VI-81. A 18-week male fetus with a complex congenital heart defect involving transposition of the great vessels and ventriculoatrial discordance. This lethal cardiac defect was diagnosed by ultrasound and led to pregnancy termination. No other developmental defects were identified; the chromosomal complement was normal; RA, right atrium; LA, left atrium; RV, right ventricle; LV, left ventricle; A, aorta; PA, pulmonary artery.

Fig. VI-82. A 19-week 45,X fetus with aortic coarctation; arrow, hypoplastic segment of aortic arch; DA, descending aorta; T, trachea; L, lungs; H, heart.

Fig. VI-83. A 19½-week 45,X female fetus with a marked hypoplasia of the ascending aorta and aortic arch (arrows); PA, pulmonary artery.

Fig. VI-84. An endocardial fibroelastosis of both the right and the left ventricle in a 16-week female fetus, which was spontaneously aborted. No myocarditis or endocarditis could be documented; nor was a viral or bacterial infection detected.

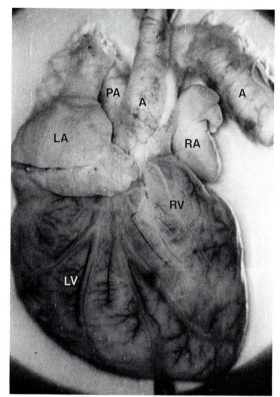

VI-81

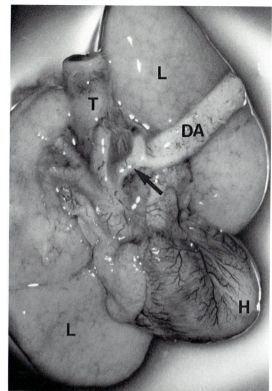

VI-82

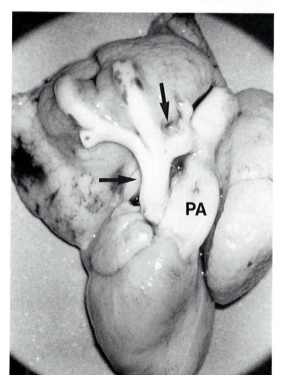

VI-83

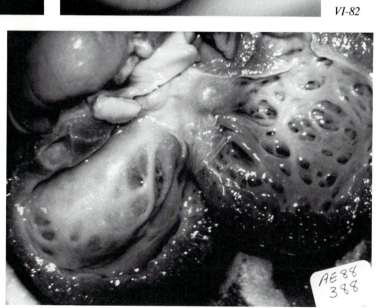

VI-84

Respiratory Tract Defects

Introduction

Among previable fetuses, the most common developmental abnormalities of the respiratory tract are the presence of abnormal fissures and/or abnormal lobation of the lungs and pulmonary hypoplasia.

Defects of the upper respiratory tract such as choanal atresia, laryngeal atresia, stenosis, and clefts are rare. *Choanal atresia* is the failure of communication between the posterior nasal sacs and the oral cavity. *Laryngeal stenosis* is a narrowing of the laryngeal cavity, and *laryngeal cleft* is incomplete formation of the larynx. Tracheoesophageal fistula is described in the next section.

Pulmonary Hypoplasia

Definition

Pulmonary hypoplasia can be assessed by the lung weight to body weight ratio, the lung volume, or a radial count. The lung volume is the most accurate (Cooney and Thurlbeck, 1985). Although lung weight represents only a crude evaluation of lung development in the previable fetus it is the most simple and practical one. Askenazi and Perlman (1979) suggest the use of lung:body weight ≤ 0.12 and a radial alveolar count ≤ 4.1 as indicative of pulmonary hypoplasia.

Embryology and Pathogenesis

At Stage 12, a median laryngotracheal groove forms on the ventral wall of the pharynx. A ridge external to the laryngotracheal groove forms and a diverticulum or tracheal bud grows from the ridge caudally and divides into the right bronchial bud and the left bronchial bud. The bronchi divide dichotomously until the end of the fourth month. Between the 10th and 14th week, 65 to 75% of the bronchial branching occurs (Brody and Thurlbeck, 1986).

Fetal pulmonary development is divided into the pseudoglandular, canalicular, and terminal sac phases (see Chapter II).

Any condition that decreases fetal respiratory movement or reduces the volume of the thorax or the amount of lung liquid will result in poor development of the lungs. Such skeletal defects as osteogenesis imperfecta, asphyxiating thoracic dystrophy, and thanatophoric dwarfism prevent normal lung development because the bone abnormalities affect both the size of the thorax and respiratory movements. Reduction of volume can also occur by compression via pleural effusion, abdominal contents in the thorax, such as in diaphragmatic hernia, or the presence of very large abdominal organs, such as polycystic kidneys. Lung development is also affected by absent or faulty innervation of the diaphragm or an absent or hypoplastic diaphragm.

Fetal lung airways are kept open by fluid derived from amniotic fluid and secretions of the tracheal and lung cells (Moore, 1977). Fetal respiratory movements move the amniotic fluid in and out of the lung, which is necessary for maturation of the lung. In oligohydramnios, the respiratory movements are decreased by external and/or internal compression. The absence or severe decrease of amniotic fluid leads to a failure to distend the air spaces. In addition, Wigglesworth et al. (1981) have suggested that normal lung secretions may not be retained within the airways in oligohydramnios.

The lungs are sometimes underdeveloped in anencephaly and other NTD. In some cases, the cause of lung hypoplasia is obvious, as in severe spinal rachischis (Brody and Thurlbeck, 1986); in other cases, the pathogenesis is not known.

Pathology

The most common cause of pulmonary hypoplasia is oligohydramnios. The histologic appearance of the lungs in oligohydramnios seems to vary. In all studies, the number of bronchi are reduced; in some studies, alveolar maturation is normal (Hislop et al., 1979); in other studies, maturation is retarded (Potter and Craig, 1975; Wigglesworth et al., 1981).

Associated Anomalies

Abnormalities unrelated to the causes or sequences of pulmonary hypoplasia are rare.

Abnormal Bronchial Division; Pulmonary Fissures and Lobes

Variations in the pattern of bronchial division are so common that they are considered normal. There may be missing or extra lobes, or there may be fissures that are partial divisions of a lobe. Particularly common are a medial accessory left lower lobe, a lateral accessory right upper lobe, and a subapical division of the lower lobes and/or the azygous lobe. The occurrence of three lobes on each side, or two lobes on each side, is often associated with heart and spleen abnormalities (Landing, 1957).

Cystic Adenomatoid Malformation of the Lung

Definition

This rare malformation is usually unilateral and often affects only one lobe. It consists of cystic structures that arise from an overgrowth of the terminal bronchioles, with a reduction in the number of alveoli. A mediastinal shift can be produced, which compresses the contralateral lung. Polyhydramnios and fetal hydrops are often present.

Pathology

Stocker divides this malformation into three types. Type I has large cysts; Type II, small cysts. Type III, the most severe type, has bronchiole-like structures separated by alveolus-like structures that occupy the entire lobe (Stocker et al., 1977).

Associated Anomalies

Renal agenesis, renal dysplasia, cardiac abnormalities, hydrocephalus, jejunal atresia, diaphragmatic hernia, bronchial abnormalities, and prune belly syndrome have been reported (Romero et al., 1988).

Pulmonary Sequestration

This rare anomaly consists of the presence of pulmonary tissue that is not attached to the rest of the lung and that does not communicate with the trachea. Where a common pleura is shared by the sequestered lung and the normal lung, this anomaly is called *intralobar pulmonary sequestration*. Intra-lobar sequestration has not been reported among previable fetuses. If a pleura is not shared, this anomaly is called *extralobar pulmonary sequestration*. Extralobar sequestration is the most common type; it is usually located between the lower lobe and the diaphragm (Romero et al., 1988). The histologic appearance of a sequestered lung may occasionally be confused with that of a cystic adenomatoid malformation. Associated anomalies are tracheoesophageal fistula, esophageal defects such as cysts, diverticula, duplications, and bronchogenic and neurogenic cysts.

Intrauterine Pneumonia

The amniotic infection syndrome described by Blanc (1959) consists of chorionitis, amnionitis, funisitis, and deglutition and inhalation of infected amniotic fluid (see Chapter VII). This may give rise to fetal infection, particularly pneumonia.

The organisms commonly involved in ascending infection are those that colonize the maternal vagina. These are usually beta hemolytic streptococci and Gram-negative bacteria, of which *Clostridium* sp. and *Escherichia coli* are most commonly isolated.

The macroscopic appearance of the infected lungs is not characteristic. They may show congestion with pleural effusion. Histologically, the lungs are edematous, congested, and inflamed. An intrauterine pulmonary infection should be distinguished from simple aspiration of infected amniotic fluid that contains maternal polymorphonuclear leukocytes. For a diagnosis of intrauterine pneumonia, the presence of peribronchial aggregates of fetal lymphocytes and polymorphonuclears within airway epithelium is required. Swab and tissue samples for bacterial cultures should always be taken to identify the pathogen.

Viral pneumonia prior to 20 weeks of gestation is a rare finding. The most commonly identified virus is cytomegalovirus. When it is seen, tiny foci of necrosis may be identified; there are also characteristic intranuclear inclusions in the surrounding viable tissue.

Fig. VI-85. Marked pulmonary hypoplasia secondary to hydrothorax and ascites in a hydropic 45,X female fetus; H, heart.

Fig. VI-86. Lungs from a 17-week male fetus with trisomy 21. The right lung shows normal lobation; note the single lobe in the left lung.

Fig. VI-87. Lungs from a 12½-week female fetus with omphalocele. The right lung shows four lobes; E, extra lobe; T, trachea.

Fig. VI-88. Lungs from a 19½-week female fetus with a normal karyotype; note the incomplete fissuration of the right lung (arrow).

Fig. VI-89. An adenomatoid malformation of the whole right lung (RL) from a 16½-week male fetus; T, trachea; LL, hypoplastic left lung.

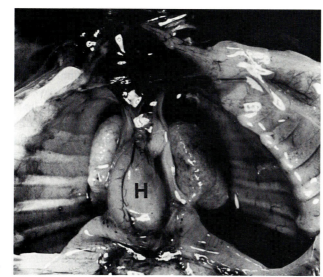

VI-85

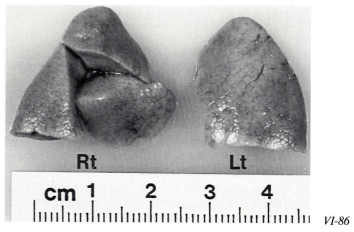

VI-86

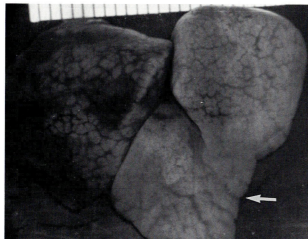

VI-88

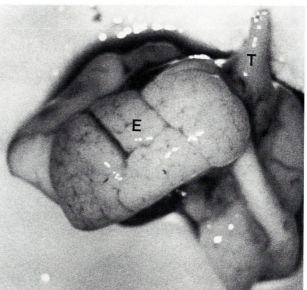

VI-87

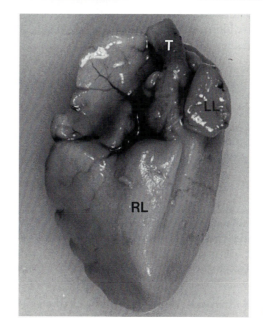

VI-89

Associated Abnormalities

Van Staey et al. (1984) reported that 45.5% of 2536 cases of esophageal atresia collected from the literature had additional congenital malformations. David and O'Callaghan (1975) reported that the most frequent malformations were gastrointestinal defects, with about one half involving an imperforate anus. The next most common defects were cardiovascular malformations, such as persistent ductus arteriosus, VSD, ASD, right-sided aortic arch, and dextrocardia. Urogenital defects, for example, renal agenesis and hydronephrosis, were the third most common associated abnormalities. Radial upper limb defects, vertebral defects, and rib defects were the most frequent types of skeletal abnormalities.

In 77 familial cases, only 21% had associated abnormalities. These were usually atresia of the duodenum or colon or an imperforate anus.

Tracheoesophageal fistula with esophageal atresia is a component of the VATER association, which is a combination of vertebral defects (V), anal atresia (A), TE fistula (TE), and radial and renal dysplasia (R).

Atresia and Stenosis of the Small Intestine

Definition

Atresia is a complete loss of continuity of the intestinal lumen; *stenosis* is a narrowing of the lumen.

Incidence

Small bowel atresias occur in approximately 1 in 5000 liveborn. The duodenum is the most common location for atresia in previable fetuses.

Embryology, Pathogenesis, and Etiology

Moutsouris (1966) described gut development in 70 normal human embryos from 7 to 40 mm in length. In the duodenum, in about two thirds of the cases, he found "moderate" epithelium proliferation; and in one third of the cases he found "considerable" epithelial proliferation, which often obliterated the lumen during the fifth week of gestation. The lumen became reestablished by the 11th week. The failure of normal recanalization is an obvious cause of duodenal atresia. The last segment to recanalize is around the ampulla of Vater, which is the usual site of duodenal obstruction (Boyden et al., 1967). In the jejunum and ileum, some degree of epithelial proliferation occurs, but complete filling of the lumen does not.

Malrotation, volvulus, intussusception, and omphalocele can cause jejunal and ileal atresia by disturbing the vascular supply to produce infarction and atrophy. In cystic fibrosis, meconium in the intestinal wall can produce obstruction with rupture, inflammation, granulation tissue, and scarring, which may lead to both atresia and stenosis.

Intestinal atresia usually is sporadic in occurrence. However, there are a few genetic forms. An autosomal recessive inheritance has been described in pyloroduodenal atresia, which is characterized by a septum between the stomach and the duodenum (Mishalany et al., 1978). Multiple bowel atresias, in which numerous atresias extend from the duodenum to the colon, is transmitted by an autosomal recessive gene (Guttman et al., 1973) and jejunal atresia (also called apple peel or Christmas tree) may also be an autosomal recessive condition (Blyth and Dickson, 1969). Trisomy 21 fetuses have duodenal atresia in less than 10%.

Pathology

There are four anatomic types of atresia. In Type I, there is a transverse septum (diaphragm) that blocks the lumen. Type II consists of blind loops of gut connected by a fibrous cord. In Type III, there is no connection between the two blind loops. In Type IV, the atretic duodenum or jejunum spirals around the vascular supply. In this apple-peel type of atresia, there is agenesis of the dorsal mesentery and absence of branches in the superior mesenteric artery.

Atresia may occur in more than one site. deLorimier et al. (1969) reviewed 613 cases of atresia and stenosis of the jejunum and ileum and found 6% multiple atresias.

Associated Abnormalities

Of patients with intestinal atresia, 50 to 70% are reported to have associated abnormalities (deLorimier et al., 1969; Fonkalsrud et al., 1969; Nixon and Tawes, 1971). However, since trisomy 21, cystic fibrosis, Hirschsprung's disease, and omphalocele are included as associated anomalies, the true incidence of associated abnormalities must be lower. In duodenal atresia, associated abnormalities other than gastrointestinal tract abnormalities are more frequent than in jejunal and ileal atresia. The most common associated abnormality in duodenal atresia is congenital heart disease, and the next most frequent is TE fistula (Fonkalsrud et al., 1969; Nixon and Tawes, 1971). The proportion of gastrointestinal abnormalities is reported higher in jejunal–ileal atresias than in duodenal stenosis.

Malrotation of the Bowel

Definition

Failure of normal rotation of the gut is called *malrotation*. This may be partial or complete.

Embryology and Pathogenesis

The normal development of the small and large intestine may be divided into three stages (Gray and Skandalakis, 1972).

The first stage is herniation. At the sixth week of gestation, the growing midgut loop enters the umbilical cord where it rotates 180° in a counterclockwise direction. The cranial (prearterial) part of the loop elongates to form more intestinal loops. In the next stage, at 10 weeks, the intestines return to the abdomen. As they return, there is a further counterclockwise rotation of 90°, so the total rotation is 270°. Most of the prearterial part of the intestine enters the abdomen first, to the right of the superior mesenteric artery. Then the colon reenters, with the cecum, and, lastly, the terminal prearterial part of the small intestine. The third stage is fixation, which continues from 11 to 12 weeks to after birth. The mesenteries

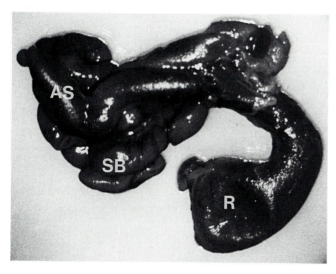

VI-92

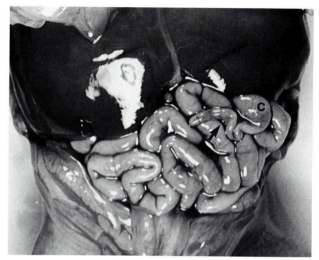

VI-94

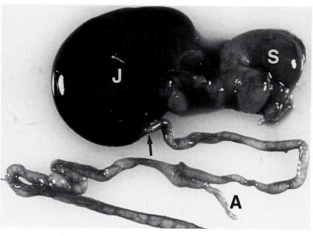

VI-93

Fig. VI-92. A short small and large bowel from a 14-week male fetus with the lethal multiple pterygium syndrome; R, rectum; AS, ascending colon; SB, small bowel. The length of the bowel is reduced to about one half the expected length for the developmental age.

Fig. VI-93. Marked dilation of the jejunum (J) is seen above the atretic segment of the small bowel (arrow); S, stomach; A, appendix. A 19-week male fetus with a normal karyotype and multiple developmental defects.

Fig. VI-94. Malrotation of the bowel in a 16-week fetus. Note the cecum (c) with the appendix (arrow) on the left side of the abdominal cavity.

of the ascending and descending parts of the intestine fuse with the parietal peritoneum, and the cecum descends to the adult position.

Most of the abnormal arrangements occur in the second stage, when the gut returns to the abdomen. In nonrotation, the colon reenters the abdomen first and lies on the left side; the cecum is in the middle and the small intestine is on the right. Vascular obstruction and volvulus may result if twisting occurs. In mixed rotation, the terminal ileum reenters the abdomen first, and the rotation is 180° instead of 270°. The cecum is subpyloric and is fixed to the abdominal wall adjacent to the duodenum. This often causes duodenal obstruction and volvulus. In reversed rotation, the first rotation is in the right direction, but only 90° instead of 180°. The second rotation is clockwise instead of counterclockwise and is 180° instead of 90°.

Failure of fixation or abnormal fixation may exert pressure on part of the intestine and obstruct its vascular supply.

Etiology

In omphalocele, since part of the intestine remains outside the abdomen, the normal pattern of entry is disturbed and this usually results in nonrotation. In diaphragmatic hernia, there is usually a nonrotation type of malrotation. In our experience, malrotation is present in about 10% of trisomy 18 and trisomy 21 fetuses. It has been reported as an occasional abnormality in the de Lange and Marfan syndromes.

Malrotation may predispose to volvulus, vascular disturbances, abnormal adhesions, and, consequently, intestinal atresia or stenosis. Biliary obstruction, an annular pancreas, and mesenteric cysts have been reported to be associated with malrotation.

Vitellointestinal Duct Remnants

The vitellointestinal (omphalomesenteric) duct is an embryonic structure that connects the embryonic gut and the yolk sac. It is normally incorporated in the connecting stalk and later obliterated. The vitelline duct may persist as a diverticulum or as a fibrous cord connecting the ileum and the umbilical area or as a cyst(s) in the umbilical cord. The persistent diverticulum is called *Meckel's diverticulum*. It is found at the terminal ileum in about 3% of normal individuals; it is more common in individuals with chromosome abnormalities. In the umbilical cord, vitellointestinal duct cysts are usually small and more prominent toward the fetal end of the cord. They are lined by the columnar, mucin-secreting epithelium and occasionally may contain pancreatic and gastric heterotopic foci.

The Short Bowel Syndrome

The normal length of the bowel at different developmental stages has been determined by Fitzsimmons et al. (1988). The bowel may be shortened in omphalocele, gastroschisis, and jejunal and ileal atresia and in fetuses in whom swallowing movements are reduced as in oligohydramnios.

Anorectal Malformations

Definition

Anorectal malformations usually refer to imperforate anus and associated abnormalities.

Incidence

Anorectal malformations occur in one to 3000 to one in 5000 live births.

Etiology

Anorectal abnormalities are found in many syndromes, as well as in some chromosomal abnormalities such as 13q⁻, trisomy 18, and cat-eye syndrome. The syndromes include dominant, recessive, and X-linked inheritance (Pinsky, 1978). Anal malformations are part of the VATER association. Maternal diabetes mellitus predisposes a fetus to anorectal abnormalities.

Embryology and Pathogenesis

At six weeks of gestation, the caudal end of the gut communicates with the allantois through the urogenital sinus. The

---

Fig. VI-95. Meckel's diverticulum (arrow) in a 10-week fetus.

Fig. VI-96. Rectal atresia (A); note the band of tissue between the rectum and the anal pit. In anal agenesis (B), the anal pit is absent. In anal stenosis (C), the anal canal is narrow.

Fig. VI-97. Anorectal abnormalities. A fistula between the rectum and vagina shown (A). The persistent cloaca (B) shows the common outlet for the rectum, vagina, and urethra. In the male, the rectum may open too anteriorly (C), or a fistula may be present between the rectum and the urethra (D).

Fig. VI-98. An external view of an imperforate anus (arrow) in a 16½-week male fetus.

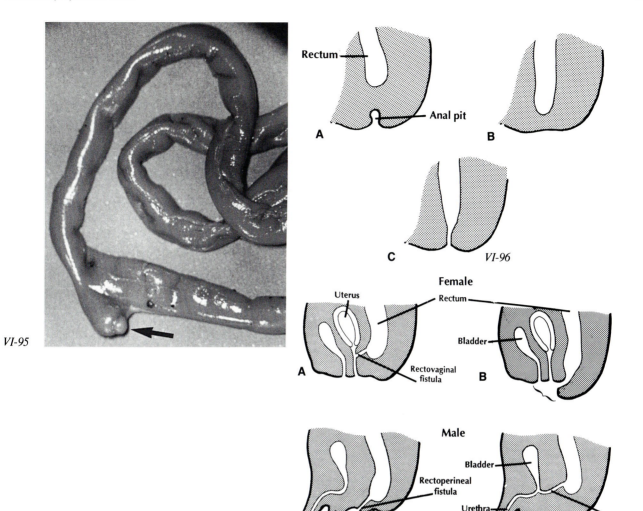

VI-95

VI-96

Female

Male

VI-97

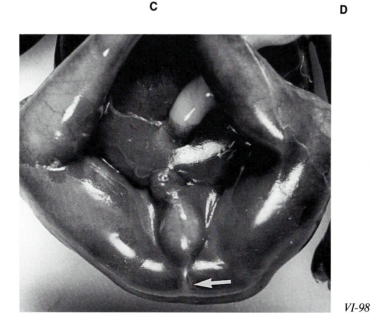

VI-98

tissue in the angle between the gut and the allantois is called the *urorectal septum*. This grows down until it reaches and fuses with the surface ectoderm. As a result of this fusion, the gut is separated from the urinary system. The tissue separating the gut and urethra from the external surface degenerates to form the urethral and anal openings. In the female, an evagination from the urogenital sinus produces most of the vagina. Further growth completely separates the vagina and the urethra.

Because of the close physical relationships of the urinary, reproductive, and gastrointestinal systems several types of fistulas involving these systems are seen. The most common are fistulas between the gut and the vagina in the female and the gut and the urethra in the male. In both cases, the gut ends blindly. The most likely cause of these abnormal communications is abnormal growth of the urogenital septum.

In normal development of the anus, the gut grows to the external surface and the ectoderm evaginates at the point of contact. Rupture of the intervening tissue produces the anal canal. An abnormality in the normal sequence of these events may result in an imperforate anus.

Pathology

Anorectal abnormalities may be high, intermediate, or low, relative to the levator ani muscle. In the male, there may be fistulas between the gut and the upper part of the urethra (rectoprostatic urethral fistula) or they may be more distal (rectobulbar urethral fistula). Another possibility is that the anus forms much closer to the penis than normal. In the female, the gut may communicate with the upper, middle, or lower portions of the vagina. In imperforate anus, the gut may terminate almost at the surface or more proximally. Prenatal diagnosis may be possible by analyzing the amniotic fluid to determine the presence or absence of certain disaccharidases (Potier et al., 1986).

Developmental Defects of the Pancreas

The pancreas is formed by two foregut buds, one dorsal and one ventral, which eventually fuse. A failure to fuse results in a division of the pancreas. Abnormal migration and fusion can produce a ring of tissue around the duodenum, the annular pancreas. Ectopic pancreatic tissue can be found in the wall of the stomach, small intestine, or Meckel's diverticulum.

Cystic Fibrosis

Definition

Cystic fibrosis is a generalized disorder of exocrine glands that is mainly characterized by pancreatic insufficiency, intestinal obstruction and chronic lung disease. The precise secretory defect in epithelial cells of the exocrine glands is not known.

Pathology

In the infant, the acini and ducts of the pancreas become distended with eosinophilic material; in the older patient, the pancreas becomes fibrotic. Mucus accumulates in the bronchi in the lung.

In the previable fetus, the pancreas and lung appear histologically normal. However, two studies of pregnancy terminations at 17 weeks for cystic fibrosis revealed that a high proportion of fetuses at this stage have a meconium ileus, as observed by Brock (1985) in all 19 of the fetuses he studied and by Muller et al. (1985) in 75% of cystic fibrotic fetuses. Because pancreatic secretions are reduced or absent, hard meconium that cannot pass the ileocecal valve is produced.

Prenatal Diagnosis

It is now possible to diagnose a majority of fetuses at risk for cystic fibrosis (Johnson, 1988). DNA is extracted from either fetal blood, amniocytes, or chorionic villi and analyzed using restriction fragment length polymorphic sites tightly linked to the locus for cystic fibrosis on chromosome 7.

Developmental Defects of the Liver

Absence of the liver is extremely rare, but accessory livers have been reported (Warkany, 1971). Ectopic liver has been noted in the abdomen and thorax. In diaphragmatic hernia, the liver may be partially in the thorax, and in ventral wall defects, the liver may protrude outside the abdomen. In these cases liver lobation is abnormal. Lobation is usually abnormal in trisomy 18 also. In polycystic disease of the kidney and in the Meckel syndrome, the liver is usually fibrotic and may be cystic. The cysts are dilations of proliferating bile ducts.

Consequences of intrahepatic or extrahepatic bile duct atresias have not been identified in previable fetuses.

Developmental Defects of the Gall Bladder

Absence of the gall bladder is usually associated with other malformations and is a common finding in fetal triploidy. The gall bladder may be completely imbedded in the liver parenchyma; therefore, careful slicing of the whole liver is required before a diagnosis of gall bladder absence can be made. Double gall bladders and a floating gall bladder (suspended from the liver by the peritoneum or mesentery) have been described (Warkany, 1971).

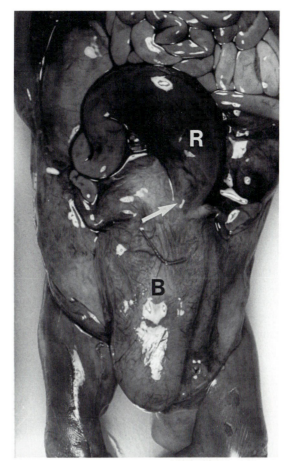

VI-99

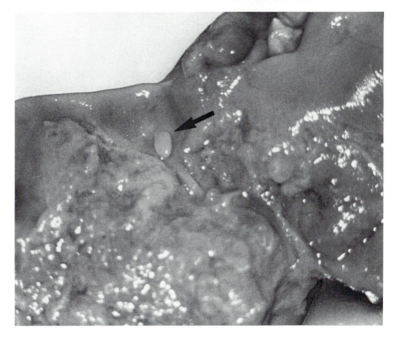

VI-100

Fig. VI-99. A rectovesical fistula (arrow) in a 16-week female fetus with agenesis of cloacal membrane. Note the dilated bladder (B), due to urethral atresia, and the dilated rectum (R).

Fig. VI-100. The inferior aspect of the degenerated liver with a hypoplastic gallbladder (arrow) in a 14-week male fetus.

Genitourinary System Defects

The Urinary System

Horseshoe Kidney

Definition

A horseshoe kidney is a single, midline, horseshoe-shaped kidney.

Incidence

Horsheshoe kidney occurs in about one in 400 to one in 600 normal individuals; it is about twice as common in males. It is a common malformation in chromosomal syndromes, especially 45,X and trisomy 13 and 18. Horseshoe kidney is also found as an occasional abnormality in some monogenic syndromes, such as Bowen-Conradi or DK-Phocomelia syndromes.

Embryology and Pathogenesis

The kidney is formed by an interaction between the ureteric bud and the metanephric blastema. If the ureteric buds are located more medially than normal or if the inducible metanephric blastema is continuous at the lower pole, then a fused horseshoe kidney may develop.

Pathology

The horseshoe kidney is usually at a lower level than normal kidneys. Its renal pelves are displaced anteriorly and its ureters usually course across the anterior surfaces of the kidney. Dysplastic development may occur in the fused portion of the kidney.

Associated Malformations

The ureters may be duplicated or angulated, so that obstruction, which leads to hydronephrosis, occurs.

Ectopic Kidney and Ureter Duplication

A kidney is *ectopic* when it is not in its usual location in the pelvis. *Ureter duplication* is a double ureter that can be unilateral or bilateral. Ectopic kidney and ureter duplication usually are not functionally important in the prenatal period. Their frequency is increased in chromosome aneuploidies.

Renal Agenesis

Definition

In renal agenesis, one or both kidneys and ureters are absent.

Incidence

Bilateral renal agenesis is rare, occurring in one in 3000 to one in 4000 liveborns. Unilateral agenesis occurs in one in 1000 newborns; it is more common in males.

Embryology and Pathogenesis

It is postulated that renal agenesis is caused by the failure of the ureteric bud, which would normally induce the metanephric blastema to become a kidney, to develop. In some cases, however, it is possible that the mesenchyme is unable to respond to the ureteric bud, which would then degenerate.

Fig. VI-101. A horseshoe kidney (H) in a 16-week, trisomy 18, male fetus with ureters (arrows) passing over the anterior aspect of the kidney; B, full urinary bladder.

Fig. VI-102. Ectopic fused hypoplastic kidneys (arrow) in a 14-week male fetus; T, testis; R, rectum.

Fig. VI-103. A duplicated right ureter (arrow) in malpositioned kidneys in a 17-week female fetus with trisomy 18.

Fig. VI-104. Renal agenesis in a 20-week male fetus; Arrows, adrenals.

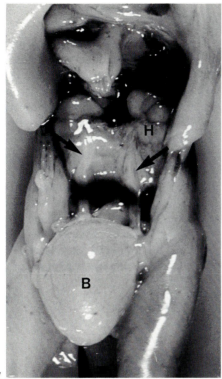

VI-101

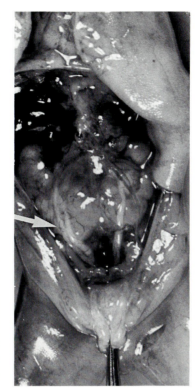

VI-103

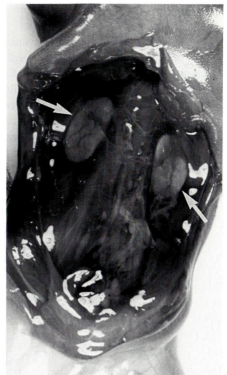

VI-104

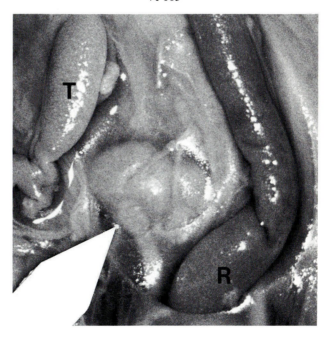

VI-102

Renal Cystic Malformations

In infantile and adult polycystic kidney disease, nephron formation and ureteric bud branching are normal. In renal dysplasia, the nephrons and ureteric bud branches are much reduced in number, and the nephrons and collecting tubules remain immature. Infantile polycystic disease and adult polycystic disease differ in their inheritance and time of onset. Infantile polycystic kidney is caused by an autosomal recessive gene and is present in the newborn. Adult polycystic kidney disease is caused by a dominant gene, and symptoms do not usually appear until the fourth decade of life.

Infantile Polycystic Kidneys

Definition

This autosomal recessive disease is characterized by bilaterally enlarged cystic kidneys. The renal lesion is usually accompanied by congenital hepatic fibrosis, with dilated hepatic bile ducts. Variation within an individual family occurs with regard to the severity of the renal and hepatic involvement.

Embryology and Pathogenesis

Hyperplasia and cystic dilation of the renal collecting ducts are attributed to an abnormal differentiation of the interstitial portion of the ureteric bud branches; the nephrons, ampulla, and pelvis are not affected.

Pathology

Bilateral involvement is characteristic. The kidneys retain their usual shape but are diffusely spongy and grossly enlarged. The collecting ducts and tubules are dilated, and there is a medullary ductal ectasia with a radial arrangement of the elongated cysts (Bernstein and Kissane, 1973). In the liver, there is portal bile ductule proliferation, sometimes accompanied by periportal fibrosis. Cysts may also be present in the lungs, pancreas, spleen, and ovary.

Associated Abnormalities

There are no associated abnormalities other than those of the oligohydramnios sequence. Infantile polycystic disease should not be confused with the cystic malformations that occur in the Meckel-Gruber syndrome or in Jeune thoracic dystrophy.

Prenatal Diagnosis

Infantile polycystic kidney can be diagnosed prenatally by ultrasound.

Fig. VI-107. (a) A 18-week male fetus with Meckel-Gruber syndrome; bilateral polycystic kidneys and polydactyly. (b) Bisected polycystic kidneys from the same fetus.

Fig. VI-108. (a) Bilateral renal dysplasia in which the parenchyma is completely replaced by cysts in a 19-week male fetus with multiple developmental defects, which include right micropthalmia, absent thumbs, absent uvula, and syndactyly in both hands and feet. The ureter and the bladder were normal. (b) Bisected kidneys show the variation in cyst size.

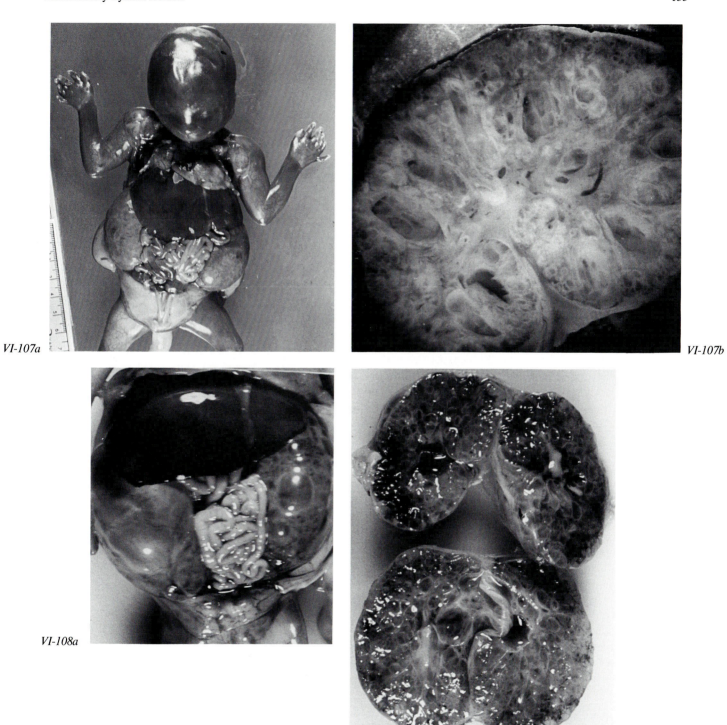

VI-107a

VI-107b

VI-108a

VI-108b

Adult Polycystic Kidney Disease

Definition

Adult polycystic disease is characterized by bilaterally enlarged kidneys. There is great variation in the severity of the disease. It may present in the newborn or remain asymptomatic through the individual's life span. Symptoms usually begin around the fourth decade of life.

Incidence

One in 1000 people have this disease.

Embryology and Pathology

Cyst size varies from millimeters to several centimeters (Bernstein and Kissane, 1973). They may be anywhere along the nephron but because they are usually due to dilation of the collecting tubules, they mainly appear there.

Associated Abnormalities

There may be cysts in other organs, such as the liver, lung, or pancreas.

Prenatal Diagnosis

A highly polymorphic DNA probe is available for prenatal diagnosis of the mutant gene on the short arm of chromosome 16 that causes dominant polycystic kidney disease. An affected fetus diagnosed by DNA studies and aborted at 12 weeks of gestation showed macroscopically normal kidneys. Microscopically, however, multiple glomerular and tubular cysts were seen in the renal cortex. The liver was microscopically normal (Reeders et al., 1986).

Renal Dysplasia

Definition

In renal dysplasia, the nephrons and ducts are immature and reduced in number. The ducts are often cystic and the number of branches of the ureter is reduced (Risdon, 1987).

Embryology and Pathogenesis

The primitive appearance of the nephrons and ducts and the reduction in nephron number and in the amount of ureter branching suggest that differentiation of the renal mesenchyme and ureter is arrested early in development. The poorly differentiated glomeruli and collecting tubules often develop cystic dilations.

Etiology

Renal dysplasia is usually sporadic and is frequently caused by a urinary outflow tract obstruction, but a few cases of familial dysplasia have been reported (Bernstein and Kissane, 1973). Renal dysplasia may be a component of syndromes, such as the Meckel-Gruber syndrome.

Pathology

Dysplastic renal development may affect the whole kidney or it may be focal or segmental. Dysplasia can be multicystic or aplastic. The multicystic dysplastic kidney is grossly cystic and enlarged. The aplastic kidney is much smaller than a normal kidney and consists of dysplastic renal tissue or small cysts.

Fig. VI-109. Unilateral renal dysplasia in a 19½-week female fetus. Note the dilated ureter and the cysts in the right kidney.

Fig. VI-110. A horseshoe kidney with hydronephrosis from a 17-week male fetus (47,XY,+13).

Fig. VI-111. A grossly dilated right ureter (arrow) and bilateral enlargement of kidneys in a 16½-week female fetus, with trisomy 13.

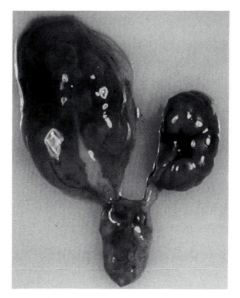

VI-109

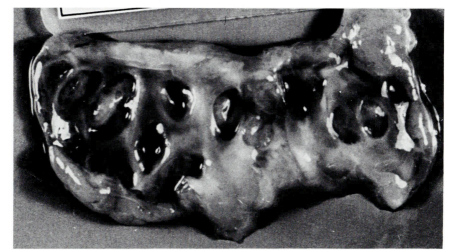

VI-110

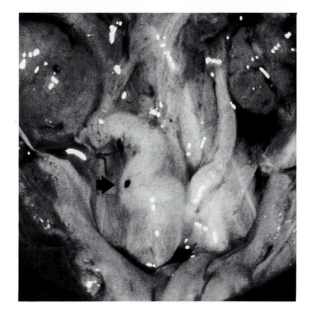

VI-111

Associated Abnormalities

Renal dysplasia is often associated with other developmental anomalies of the urinary tract. Bilateral renal dysplasia occurs in the oligohydramnios sequence. Unilateral renal dysplasia may be associated with such other major developmental defects as isolated ventricular septal defect, aortic coarctation, intestinal atresia, or meningomyelocele (Risdon, 1987).

Hydronephrosis

Definition

In this condition, the renal pelvis is dilated and some of the renal parenchyma may be atrophied due to the obstruction of the ureters or urethra and subsequent dysplastic development.

Pathogenesis and Etiology

Obstruction of the pathway of urine flow is the cause of hydronephrosis, although it is not always possible to determine the location or to identify the cause of the obstruction. Ureteropelvic junction obstruction is the most common cause of fetal hydronephrosis. Pressure on the ureter by an aberrant blood vessel may also reduce urine flow. Ureter muscle abnormalities, such as sparseness and fibrosis (Tokunaka et al., 1984a), have been reported as other causes of reduced urine flow. Bladder diverticula adjacent to the ureter orifice might also cause obstruction (Tokunaka et al., 1980b), as might posterior urethral valves and urethral maldevelopment.

Pathology

The pelvicalyceal area is dilated and the renal parenchyma is atrophied. The severity of renal atrophy depends on the degree of obstruction and the length of time it has been present.

Associated Abnormalities

There may be abnormalities of the urinary tract other than those that cause hydronephrosis. Hydronephrosis is part of the prune belly syndrome and the megacystis–microcolon–intestinal hypoperistalsis syndrome (Romero et al., 1988). In this latter syndrome, there is a large thin bladder, a hydroureter, and hydronephrosis, and the kidneys are often dysplastic. About 30% of cases of campomelic dysplasia have hydronephrosis, and it is occasionally present in thanatophoric dwarfism and dyssegmental dysplasia.

Posterior Urethral Valves

Definition

Valvular folds of the urethral mucous membrane normally occur only in the male.

There are three types of valvular folds, but only Types I and III can cause obstruction. In Type I, the two folds that are normally present and that extend from the verumontanum into the lateral wall of the urethra are enlarged and block urine outflow. In Type II, the folds extend posteriorly from the upper edge of the verumontanum without causing obstruction. In Type III, a transverse diaphragm blocks the urethra distal to the verumontanum.

Embryology and Pathogenesis

Folds are normally present in the male urethra, but they are not large enough to cause blockage. In Type I, there seems to be an overgrowth of the folds, with a possible abnormal insertion of the distal end of the Wolffian duct (Romero et al., 1988). The transverse diaphragm seen in Type III folds may be related to a defect of the urogenital membrane.

Etiology

Although posterior urethral valves are almost always spo-

Fig. VI-112. (a) A 19-week male fetus with a large distended abdomen due to urethral atresia and urinary bladder dilation. Note the clubbing of both feet. (b) The same fetus, with a markedly dilated urinary bladder (UB) and ureters (arrows). The kidneys are dilated and cystic.

Fig. VI-113. (a) A macerated 19-week male fetus with a distended abdomen and clubfeet. The abdominal distension is due to a posterior urethral valve that has produced a dilated bladder, hydroureters, and early cystic changes in both kidneys. (b) The same fetus, showing a dilated urinary bladder (UB) and hydroureters (arrows).

Fig. VI-114. A 10½-week male fetus with hypospadia (arrow).

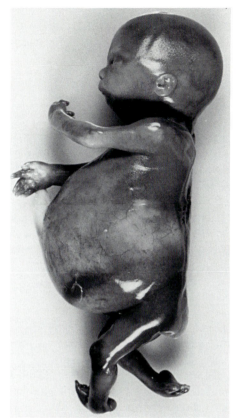

VI-112a

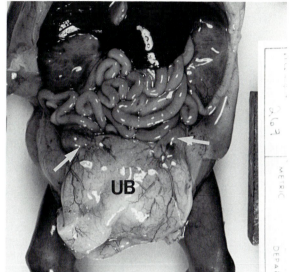

VI-112b

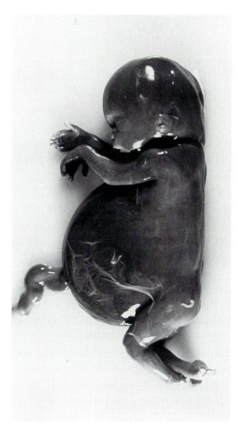

VI-113a

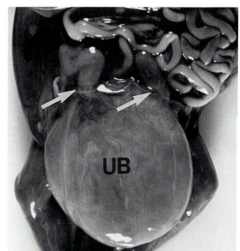

VI-113b

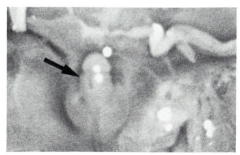

VI-114

radic, there have been two reports of familial posterior urethral valves (Davidsohn and Newberger, 1933; Hasen and Song, 1955).

Pathology

Obstruction of the urethra can produce enlargement and hypertrophy of the bladder and hydroureters, and bilateral hydronephrosis. Renal dysplasia due to renal damage may be observed if the obstruction occurs early in development.

Associated Abnormalities

Abnormalities of the genitourinary tract, such as duplication of the urethra, hypospadias, and cryptorchidism, are commonly seen in obstructive uropathies due to posterior urethreal valves. Other abnormalities reported are imperforate anus, skeletal anomalies, and heart and blood vessel abnormalities. Posterior urethral valves may occur in the prune belly syndrome.

Prune Belly Sequence

Definition

The prune belly sequence, or syndrome consists of urinary tract abnormalities, cryptorchidism, and an abdominal muscle deficiency. Almost all cases are males.

Incidence

The prune belly sequence occurs in one in 3500 to one in 5000 liveborn.

Embryology and Pathogenesis

Prune belly refers to a thin redundant abdominal skin, which some people think resembles a prune. This appearance is due to anterior abdominal wall muscle deficiency. This deficiency may occasionally be a primary muscle defect, but in most cases it seems to be secondary to abdominal distension caused by a dilated hypertrophic urinary bladder. The vast majority of cases occurs in males, and since the kidneys, ureters, and bladder always show the consequences of obstruction, it is thought that abnormalities of the urethra are the main cause (Pagon et al., 1979a).

Etiology

Prune belly sequence is usually sporadic. It has been reported in trisomy 13 and 18 and in 45,X.

Pathology

It is important to search for the cause of obstruction, since different types of urethral obstruction have been described (Wigger and Blanc, 1977). There may be atresia, posterior urethral valves, stenosis, or even urethral absence. The prostate may be hypoplastic. In some cases, no cause of urethral obstruction can be determined. The bladder is usually dilated and may be hypertrophic; the ureters are dilated; and the kidneys may be hydronephrotic and/or dysplastic.

Associated Abnormalities

Skeletal anomalies, especially of the rib cage, are common and cardiovascular abnormalities, cleft palate, and unilateral renal agenesis have also been reported.

Gut malrotation and cryptorchidism are often present. The bladder distension may interfere with gut rotation and testes descent. It may also compress the blood vessels and cause lower limb deficiencies.

The Genital System

Normal Development

In the four-week embryo, the genital ridge forms medial to the mesonephros. The germ cells, at first in the wall of the yolk sac, migrate towards the genital ridges and enter them at six weeks of gestation. The epithelium of the genital ridge by then has proliferated into a network, the primitive sex cords, in which the germ cells are found. Since males and females are indistinguishable at this time, it is called the *indifferent gonad stage.*

The embryonic gonad is intrinsically programmed to become an ovary. If a gene(s) that produces testis-determining factor (TDF) is present, the gonad will start to develop into a testis between six and eight weeks. Leydig cells and Sertoli cells begin to differentiate within the testes. The Leydig cells produce testosterone, which stimulates further development of the seminal vesicle, vas deferens, and epididymis. A derivative of testosterone, dihydrotestosterone, induces differentiation of the penis, scrotum, and prostate. The Sertoli cells produce the Müllerian inhibiting factor, which causes the Müllerian ducts to regress. The Sertoli cells start to secrete at 45 to 50 days; the Leydig cells at about 60 days. If the indifferent gonad has not been exposed to TDF by eight to nine weeks, the gonad can no longer respond by becoming a testis.

The external genitalia look the same in both sexes at six weeks of development to eight.

In the female, germ cells are found in primordial ovarian follicles, which develop at the epithelial side of the gonad that has become an ovary by the seventh week of development. The female external genitalia start to develop at the eighth week.

Only the most common abnormalities of the male and female reproductive system are listed here (Saenger, 1984; Simpson, 1976, 1983; Pinsky and Kaufman, 1987). Abnormalities of the genital system are divided into those with external manifestations, and those with internal abnormalities.

Abnormal External Genitalia

The most common male abnormalities are hypospadias and small penis. Females with an enlarged clitoris are included in the ambiguous genitalia.

Ambiguous genitalia are rarely found in the previable period. The most common causes of ambiguous sexual development are summarized in Table VI-8. It is obvious from the table that the karyotype of the fetus must be known for proper evaluation.

Sometimes the karyotype does not correspond to the appearance of the external genitalia. Table VI-9 lists some conditions in which this occurs.

Abnormal Internal Reproductive Tracts

Defects in the internal reproductive tracts are rare as isolated findings. They are usually found as a component of a complex malformation syndrome, such as sirenomelia. In female fetuses with a normal female karyotype, abnormalities of the internal reproductive tract include absent ovary, ovary showing gonadal dysgenesis, and Müllerian aplasia consisting of atresias, fistulas, and abnormal septa.

In male fetuses with a normal male karyotype, anorchia and Wolffian aplasia can be seen.

TABLE VI.8. Ambiguous external genitalia.

1. Normal male karyotype with no other anomalies

Male	*Female*
Abnormal testosterone synthesis	Excess androgens
deficiency of	
cholesterol desmolase	3 β hydroxysteroid
3 β hydroxysteroid	dehydrogenase
dehydrogenase	deficiency
17 α-hydroxylase	21 hydroxylase deficiency
17,20 desmolase	11 hydroxylase deficiency
17-hydroxysteroid	Maternal androgen or
dehydrogenese	progestin ingestion
Abnormal testosterone	
metabolism	Tumors producing excess
5α reductase deficiency	of androgenes
XY gonadal dysgenesis	
(some)	
Agonadia (absent testis)	

2. Normal karyotype with multiple associated anomalies
      Many syndromes

3. Abnormal karyotypes
      45,X/46,XY:
      46,XX/46,XY
      45,X/47,XYY
      46,XX/47,XXY
      Many syndromes

TABLE VI.9. Discordance between external genitalia and karyotype.

Female external genitalia with XY karyotype
   Androgen insufficiency syndromes
   XY gonadal dysgenesis (some)
   Leydig cell agenesis

Male external genitalia with XX karyotype
   XX Males
   True hermaphrodites (some)

In previable female fetuses with an abnormal X chromosome, there are usually no morphologic defects. The Müllerian ducts are well differentiated and the ovaries appropriately developed for the gestational age. Loss of ova and an increase in fibrous tissue usually occur after 20 weeks of gestation.

For gonad descriptions in 47,XXY and 47,XYY fetuses, see Chapter IX.

AMNION RUPTURE SEQUENCE AND LIMB BODY WALL COMPLEX

Introduction

We have divided amnion defects into the limb body wall complex (LBWC), caused by an early defect in the amniotic sac, and the amnion rupture sequence (ARS), caused by amniotic bands. Although their etiology and pathogenesis is not known, the defects seem to appear at different developmental stages.

The LBWC defect probably occurs (Van Allen et al., 1987) at an early embryonic stage (3 to 6 weeks gestation) when there is an intimate relationship between the amniotic sac and the embryo long before the amnion and chorion have fused. The affected embryo/fetus usually has large defects involving the lateral body wall and/or facial cleft(s), with cranial and limb defects. In the LBWC, the amnion is continuous with the margin of the body wall defect or the cranial defect, and the body stalk is very short.

The ARS probably occurs later when the body wall and neural tube are closed. The nature of the fetal defects mainly depends on the location of the amniotic bands attached to the fetus and their interference with normal embryonic/fetal development.

Amnion Rupture Sequence

Definition

Amnion rupture sequence refers to the damage caused to the fetus by amniotic bands that are the result of amnion tear. Amniotic bands may interfere with normal embryonic development to cause malformations, deformations, or disruptions. Amnion rupture may also cause a loss of amniotic fluid and produce secondary effects on fetal development due to oligohydramnios.

The severity of fetal malformations, disruptions, and deformations vary greatly. Multiple synonyms have been used to describe the ARS. These have been summarized by Seed et al.

(1982) and include aberrant tissue bands, ADAM complex, amniogenic bands, amniotic band disruption complex, amniotic band syndrome, and congenital annular bands or constrictions.

Incidence

In a study of 1010 previable fetuses, an incidence of one in 56 cases was reported (Kalousek and Bamforth, 1988). This is a much higher incidence than the one in 2500 newborns reported by Ossipof and Hall (1977).

Embryology and Pathogenesis

The amniotic cavity develops by day eight as a slit-like space between the embryonic disc and the trophoblast. It continues to enlarge to encompass the developing embryo, but not until 12 postconceptional weeks does the amnion fuse with the chorion. The cavity is lined by amnioblasts that probably have arisen from both cytotrophoblast and embryonic epiblasts.

Based on an evaluation of fetal defects caused by amniotic bands, it is clear that they occur at different times. Cases with neural tube defects (anencephaly or encephalocele) and/or facial defects (irregular clefts) indicate the presence of amniotic bands interfering with the normal sequence of embryonic development before 40 days of development. Disruptions and deformations of structures that had previously developed normally, for example, amputation of digits or limbs, indicate a later effect.

Although the etiology of amniotic bands is not known, abdominal trauma, amniocentesis, and connective tissue abnormalities (Young et al., 1985; Van der Rest et al., 1986) have been suggested as possible causes. In most cases, however, there is no such associated event.

Pathology

Amniotic bands can be demonstrated during the embryonic period as fine bands of amnion. Although they are much finer than the bands commonly observed during the fetal period,

---

Fig. VI-117. An embryo (Stage 17) with an amniotic band around a limb bud (arrow).

Fig. VI-118. A 10½-week male fetus. Note the amniotic bands causing finger and toe amputations and constrictions; C, constriction of the umbilical cord.

Fig. VI-119. A 14-week fetus with a band around the left ankle (arrows) and amputated distal phalanges of three toes.

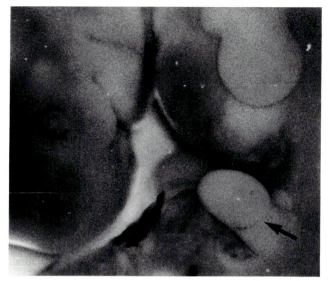

VI-117

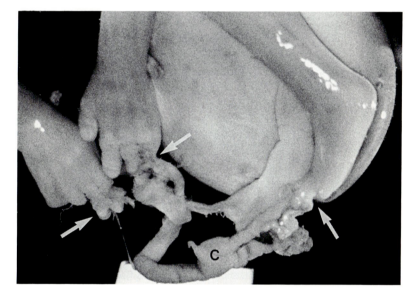

VI-118

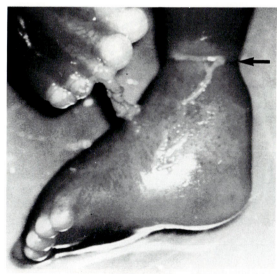

VI-119

filled with a proteinaceous fluid, which can be of either low or high viscosity. Numerous dilated lymph channels are usually seen in the walls of the cavities in cystic hygromas of non-45,X fetuses, whereas 45,X fetuses show only occasional lymphatic vessels (Chitayat et al., 1989). The same difference in number of lymph vessels exists in other parts of the body, specifically, the limbs.

Advances in sonography has allowed accurate prenatal detection of fetal cystic hygroma (Chervenak et al., 1983). If the decision is made to terminate the pregnancy, every effort should be made to determine the cause of the cystic hygroma. Most cases are found to be monosomy X; however, this diagnosis should be supported by chromosome analysis. When amniocentesis is not done or when the fetal tissue culture fails to grow, one must rely on fetal autopsy findings.

Kalousek and Seller (1987) found that all 61 previable fetuses with monosomy X have a triad of morphologic findings: nuchal cystic hygroma, generalized edema, and aortic coarctation. Recognition of this triad can aid in making the diagnosis of monosomy X when chromosome analysis is not available. When the specimen is fragmented or incomplete, however, the only way to support a diagnosis of 45,X is by a histopathologic study to show cutaneous edema with peripheral lymphatic hypoplasia.

References

Aitken J: Exomphalos. *Arch Dis Child* 38:126–129, 1963.

Allan L, Crawford D, Chita S, Anderson R, Tynan M: Familial recurrence of congenital heart disease in a prospective series of mothers referred for fetal echocardiography. *Am J Cardiol* 58:334–337, 1986.

Anderson RH, Allan L: The heart. In *Diseases of the Fetus and Newborn*, Reed GB, Claireaux AE, Bain AD (eds): London, Chapman and Mall Medical, 1989, pp 217–241.

Askenazi S, Perlman M: Pulmonary hypoplasia: Lung weight and radial alveolar count as criteria of diagnosis. *Arch Dis Child* 54:614–618, 1979.

Baird P, MacDonald E: An epidemiologic study of congenital malformations of the anterior abdominal wall in more than half a million consecutive live births. *Am J Hum Genet* 33:470–478, 1981.

Bartsocas C, Papas C: Popliteal pterygium syndrome. *J Med Genet* 9:222–226, 1972.

Becker AE, Anderson RH: *Pathology of Congenital Heart Disease.* London, Butterworths, 1981.

Becker AE, Anderson RH: *Cardiac Pathology—An Integrated Text and Colour Atlas.* London, Gower Medical Publishing, 1983.

Beckwith J: Macroglossia, omphalocele, adrenal cytomegaly, gigantism, and hyperplastic visceromegaly. *Birth Defects* 5(2):188, 1969.

Bell J: The pathology of central nervous system defects in human fetuses of different gestational ages, in Persaud (ed): *Central Nervous System and Craniofacial Malformations, Advances in the Study of Birth Defects.* New York, Alan R. Liss, Inc., 1982, vol 7, p 10.

Benacerraf B, Adzick N: Fetal diaphragmatic hernia: Ultrasound diagnosis and clinical outcome in 19 cases. *Am J Obstet Gynecol* 156:573–576, 1987.

Bernstein J, Kissane J: Hereditary Disorders of the Kidney, in Rosenberg N, Bolande R (eds): *Perspectives in Pediatric Pathology.* Chicago, Year Book Medical Publishers, vol 1, 1973, p 117.

Bieber F, Petres R, Bleber J, Nance W: Prenatal detection of a familial nuchal bleb simulating encephalocele. *Birth Defects* OAS XV no 5A 51–61, 1979.

Biedel C, Pagon R, Zapata J: Müllerian anomalies and renal agenesis: Autosomal dominant urogenital adysplasia. *J Pediat* 104:861, 1984.

Blanc W: Amniotic infection syndrome: Pathogenesis, morphology and significance in circumnatal mortality. *Clin Obstet Gynecol* 2:705–734, 1959.

Blyth H, Dickson J: Apple peel syndrome. *J Med Genet* 6:275–277, 1969.

Bonham Carter R, Waterston D, Aberdeen E: Hernia and eventration of the diaphragm in childhood. *Lancet* i:656–659, 1962.

Boyden E, Cope J, Bill A: Anatomy and embryology of congenital intrinsic obstruction of the duodenum. *Am J Surg* 114:190–202, 1967.

Brock D: A comparative study of microvillar enzyme activities in the prenatal diagnosis of cystic fibrosis. *Prenat Diag* 5:129–134, 1985.

Brody J, Thurlbeck W: Development, growth, and aging of the lung, in *Handbook of Physiology*, Section 3. *The Respiratory System*, vol 3. Baltimore, Williams & Wilkins, 1986, pp 355–376.

Burn J: Commentary. *Br J Obstet Gynecol* 94:97–99, 1987.

Byrne J, Warburton D: Neural tube defects in spontaneous abortions. *Am J Med Genet* 25:327–333, 1986.

Byrne J, Blanc W, Warburton D, Wigger J: The significance of cystic hygroma in fetuses. *Hum Pathol* 15:61–67, 1984.

Byrne J, Warburton D, Kline J, Blanc W, Stein Z: Morphology of

---

Fig. VI-135. A 16-week 46,XX female with tetralogy of Fallot, generalized edema, and ascites; posterior cervical hygroma shows anterior extension (arrow).

Fig. VI-136. A 17-week 46,XX female with a cystic cervical hygroma and no other anomalies.

Fig. VI-137. A 16-week 46,XX male with mild subcutaneous posterior cervical edema. This was diagnosed as a cystic hygroma on ultrasound examination.

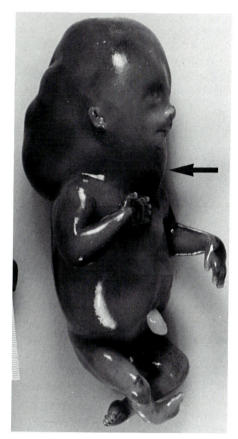

VI-135

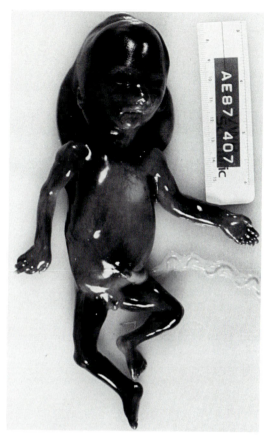

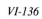

VI-136

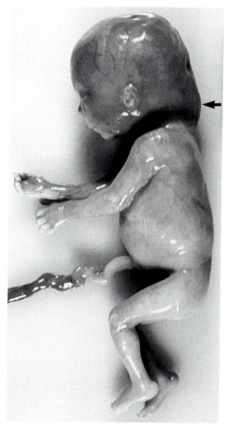

VI-137

early fetal deaths and their chromosomal characteristics. *Teratology* 32:297–315, 1985.

Campbell L, Dayton D, Sohal G: Neural tube defects: A review of human and animal studies of the etiology of neural tube defects. *Teratology* 34:171–187, 1986.

Cantrell J, Haller J, Ravitch M: A syndrome of congenital defects involving the abdominal wall, sternum, diaphragm, pericardium and heart. *Surg Gynecol Obstet* 107:602–614, 1958.

Carey J, Greenbaum B, Hall B: The OEIS complex (omphalocele, extrophy, imperforate anus, spinal defects). *Birth Defects* OAS XIV, 6B, 253–263, 1978.

Chen H, Immken L, Lachman R, Yang S, Rimoin D, Rightmire D, Eteson D, Stewart F, Beemer F, Opitz J, Gilbert E, Langer L, Shapiro L, Duncan P: Syndrome of multiple pterygia, camptodactyly, facial anomalies, hypoplastic lung and heart, cystic hygroma and skeletal anomalies. *Am J Med Genet* 17:809–826, 1984.

Chervenak F, Isaacson G, Blakemore K, Breg W, Hobbins J, Berkewitz R, Tortora M, Mayden K, Mahoney M: Fetal cystic hygroma. *New Engl J Med* 309:822–825, 1983.

Chervenak F, Isaacson G, Hobbins J, Chitkara U, Tortora M, Berkowitz R: Diagnosis and management of fetal holoprosencephaly. *Obstet Gynecol* 6:322–326, 1985.

Chitayat D, Kalousek D, Bamforth J: The lymphatic abnormalities in fetuses with posterior cervical cystic hygroma. *Am J Med Genet* 33:352–356, 1989.

Clark S, DeVore G, Sabey P: Prenatal diagnosis of cysts of the fetal choroid plexus. *Obstet Gynecol* 72:585–586, 1988.

Cohen M: An update on the holoprosencephalic disorders. *J Pediatr* 101:865–869, 1982.

Cohen M: Craniofacial disorders, in Emery A, Rimoin D (eds): *Principles and Practice of Medical Genetics.* Edinburgh, Churchill Livingstone, 1983, pp 576–622.

Cohen M: Perspectives on holoprosencephaly: Part III. Spectra, distinctions, continuities and discontinuities. Am J Med Genet 34:271–288, 1989.

Cohen M, Lemire R: Syndromes with cephaloceles. *Teratology* 25:161–172, 1982.

Cooney T, Thurlbeck W: Lung growth and development in anencephaly and hydrancephaly. *Am Rev Respir Dis* 132:596–601, 1985.

Cowchock F, Wapner R, Kurtz A, Chatzkel S, Barnhart J, Lesnick D: Brief clinical report: Not all cystic hygromas occur in the Ullrich–Turner syndrome. *Am J Med Genet* 12:327–331, 1982.

Creasy M, Alberman E: Congenital malformations of the central nervous system in spontaneous abortions. *J Med Genet* 13:9–16, 1976.

Czeizel A, Vitez M: Etiological study of omphalocele. *Hum Genet* 58:390–395, 1981.

David T, Illingworth C: Diaphragmatic hernia in the southwest of England. *J Med Genet* 13:253–262, 1976.

David T, O'Callaghan S: Oesophageal atresia in the southwest of England. *J Med Genet* 12:1–11, 1975.

David T, Nixon A: Congenital malformations associated with anencephaly and iniencephaly. *J Med Genet* 13:263–265, 1976.

Davidsohn I, Newberger C: Congenital valves of the posterior urethra in twins. *Arch Pathol* 16:57–62, 1933.

Davis J, Kalousek D: Fetal akinesia deformation sequence in previable fetuses. *Am J Med Genet* 29:77–87, 1988.

Dekaban A, Bartelmez G: Complete dysraphism in 14 somite human embryo. *Am J Anat* 115:27–42, 1964.

DeLange S: Progressive hydrocephalus, in Vinken P, and Bruyn G (eds): *Congenital Malformations of the Brain and Skull. Handbook of Clinical Neurology,* Amsterdam, Elsevier North Holland Publishing Co, 1977, vol 30, p 525.

deLorimier A, Fonkalsrud E, Hays D: Congenital atresia and stenosis of the jejunum and ileum. *Surgery* 65:819–827, 1969.

deVries P: The pathogenesis of gastroschisis and omphalocele. *J Pediatr Surg* 15:245–251, 1980.

Demyer W: Holoprosencephaly, in Vinken P, and Bruyn G (eds): *Congenital Malformations of the Brain and Skull. Handbook of Clinical Neurology,* Elsevier North Holland Publishing Co, Amsterdam, 1977, vol 30, p 431.

Dodds G, DeAngelis E: An anencephalic embryo 16.5 mm long. *Anat Rec* 67:499–505, 1937.

Dorovini-Zis K, Dolman CL: Gestational development of the brain. *Arch Pathol Lab Med* 101:192–198, 1977.

Dott N: Clinical record of case of exomphalos, illustrating embryonic type and its surgical treatment. *Trans Edinburgh Obstet Soc* 52:105–108, 1932.

Duhamel B: From the mermaid to anal imperforation: The syndrome of caudal regression. *Arch Dis Child* 36:152–155, 1961.

Fitzsimmons J, Chinn A, Shepard T: Normal length of the human fetal gastrointestinal tract. *Pediatr Pathol* 8:663–641, 1988.

Fonkalsrud E, deLorimier A, Hays D: Congenital atresia and stenosis of the duodenum. *Pediatrics* 43:79–83, 1969.

Fraser FC, Nussbaum E: Neural tube defects in sibs of children with tracheo-esophageal dysraphism. *Lancet* ii:807, 1980.

Fryns J, Moerman F, Goddeeris P, Bossuyt C, Van den Berghe H: A new lethal syndrome with cloudy cornea, diaphragmatic defects and distal limb deformities. *Hum Genet* 50:65–70, 1979.

Gellis S, Feingold M: Caudal dysplasia syndrome. *Am J Dis Child* 116:407–408, 1968.

Gilbert W, Nicolaides K: Fetal omphalocele: Associated malformations and chromosomal defects. *Obstet Gynecol* 70:633–635, 1987.

Gillin M, Pryse-Davis J: Case report. Pterygium syndrome. *J Med Genet* 13:249–251, 1976.

Graham J, Smith D: Dominantly inherited pterygium colli. *J Pediatr* 98:664–665, 1981.

Gray S, Skandalakis J: *Embryology for Surgeons.* Philadelphia, Saunders, 1972, p 129.

Greenwood R, Rosenthal A, Nadas A: Cardiovascular malformations associated with omphalocele. *J Pediatr* 85:818–821, 1974.

Greenwood R, Rosenthal A, Nadas A: Cardiovascular abnormalities associated with congenital diaphragmatic hernia. *Pediatrics* 57:92–97, 1976.

Guttman F, Braun P, Garance P, Blanchard H, Collin P, Dallaire L, Desjardins J, Perreault G: Multiple atresias and a new syndrome of hereditary multiple atresias involving the gastrointestinal tract from stomach to rectum. *J Pediatr Surg* 8:633–640, 1973.

Hall J: Invited Editorial Comment: Analysis of Pena Shokeir phenotype. *Am J Med Genet* 25:99–117, 1986.

Hall J, Reed S, Rosenbaum J, Gershanik J, Chen H, Wilson K: Limb pterygium syndromes. *Am J Med Genet* 12:377–409, 1982.

Hall J, Friedman J, Keena B, Popkin J, Jawanda M, Arnold W: Clinical, genetic and epidemiological factors in neural tube defects. *Am J Hum Genet* 43:827–837, 1988.

Hamilton W, Boyd J, Mossman H: *Human Embryology.* 4th edition. Baltimore, Williams & Wilkins, 1978.

Hansen J, James S, Burrington J, Whitfield J: The decreasing incidence of pneumothorax and improving survival of infants with congenital diaphragmatic hernia. *J Pediatr Surg* 19:385–388, 1984.

Hasen H, Song Y: Congenital valvular obstruction of the posterior urethra in two brothers. *J Pediatr* 47:207–215, 1955.

Havalad S, Noblett H, Speidel B: Familial occurrence of omphalocele suggesting sex-linked inheritance. *Arch Dis Child* 54:142–151, 1979.

Herva R, Karkinen-Jaaskelainen M: Amniotic adhesion malformation syndrome. Fetal and placental pathology. *Teratology* 29:11–19, 1984.

Herva R, Leisti J, Kirkinen P, Seppanen U: A lethal autosomal recessive syndrome of multiple congenital contractures. *Am J Med Genet* 20:431–439, 1985.

Hislop A, Hey E, Reid L: The lungs in congenital bilateral renal agenesis and dysplasia. *Arch Dis Child* 54:32–38, 1979.

Ho SY, Wilcox BR, Anderson RH, Lincoln JCR: Interrupted aortic arch – anatomic features of surgical significance. *Thorac Cardiovasc Surg* 31:199–205, 1983.

Holden M, Wooler G: Tracheo-oesophageal fistula and oesophageal atresia: Results of 30 years' experience. *Thorax* 25:406–412, 1970.

Hoyme H, Higginbottom M, Jones K: The vascular pathogenesis of gastrochisis: Intrauterine interruption of the omphalomesenteric artery. *J Pediatr* 98:228–231, 1981.

Isaacson G, Gargus J, Mahoney M: Lethal multiple pterygium syndrome in an 18-week fetus with hydrops. *Am J Med Genet* 17:835–839, 1984.

Johnson J: Genetic counseling used linked DNA probes: Cystic fibrosis as a prototype. *J Pediatr* 113:957–964, 1988.

Jones K: *Smith's Recognizable Patterns of Human Malformations*, Ed 4, Philadelphia, WB Saunders, 1988.

Kallen B: Overgrowth malformation and neoplasia in embryonic brain. Confin Neurol 22:40–60, 1962.

Kalousek D: The role of confined placental mosaicism in placental function and human development. *Growth Genet Horm* 4:1–3, 1988.

Kalousek DK, Bamforth S: Amnion rupture sequence in previable fetuses. *Am J Med Genet* 31:63–73, 1988.

Kalousek D, Seller M: Differential diagnosis of posterior cervical hygroma in previable fetuses. *Am J Med Genet* (Suppl 3):83–92, 1987.

Kampmeier O: On sireniform monsters with a consideration of the causation and predominance of the male sex among them. *Anat Rec* 34:365–388, 1927.

Keeling JW (ed): Fetal hydrops, in Keeling JW (ed): *Fetal and Neonatal Pathology*, Berlin Heidelberg New York, Springer-Verlag, 1987, pp 211–228.

Keeling J (ed): *Fetal and Neonatal Pathology*. Berlin Heidelberg New York, Springer-Verlag, 1987.

Keeling JW, Gough DJ, Iliff P: The pathology of non-Rhesus hydrops. *Diagn Histopathol* 6:89–111, 1983.

Khoury M, Erickson J, James L: Etiologic heterogeneity of neural tube defects: Clues from epidemiology. *Am J Epidemiol* 115:538–548, 1982.

Kallen B: Overgrowth malformation and neoplasia in embryonic brain. *Confin Neurol* 22:40–60, 1962.

Landing B: in Nelson (ed): *Pediatric Clinics of North America*. Philadelphia, WB Saunders, 1957, p 73.

Laurence K: Hydrocephalus and malformations of the central nervous system, in Keeling JW (ed): *Fetal and Neonatal Pathology*. Berlin Heidelberg New York, Springer-Verlag, 1987, p 463.

Lemire R, Beckwith J, Warkany J: *Anencephaly*. New York, Raven Press, 1978.

Lemire R, Cohen M, Beckwith J, Kokich V, Siebert J: The facial features of holoprosencephaly in anencephalic human specimens. *Teratology* 23:297–303, 1981.

Leong A, Shaw C: The pathology of occipital encephalocele and a discussion of the pathogenesis. *Pathology* 11:223–234, 1979.

Lorber J: The prognosis of occipital encephalocele. *Dev Med Child Neural* [Suppl] 13:75–86, 1966.

Mall FP: A study of the causes underlying the origin of human monsters. *J Morphol* 19:3–368, 1908.

Mann L, Ferguson-Smith M, Desai M, Gibson A, Raine P: Prenatal assessment of anterior abdominal wall defects and their prognosis. *Prenatal Diag* 4:427–435, 1984.

McFadden D, Kalousek D: Survey of neural tube defects in spontaneously aborted embryos. *Am J Med Genet* 32:356–358, 1989.

McKeown T, MacMahon B, Record R: An investigation of 69 cases of exomphalos. *Am J Hum Genet* 5:168–175, 1953.

MacHenry J, Nevin N, Merrett J: Comparison of central nervous system malformations in spontaneous abortions in Northern Ireland and Southeast England. *Br Med J* 1:1395–1397, 1979.

Matsunaga E, Shiota K: Holoprosencephaly in human embryos: Epidemiologic studies of 150 cases. *Teratology* 16:261–272, 1977.

Mishalany H, Idriss Z, der Kaloustian V: Pyloroduodenal atresia (diaphragm type): An autosomal recessive disease. *Pediatrics* 62:419–421, 1978.

Moerman P, Fryns J, Devlieger H, Van Assche A, Lauweryns J: Congenital eventration of the diaphragm. *Am J Med Genet* 27:213–218, 1987.

Moessinger A: Fetal akinesia deformation sequence: an animal model. *Pediatrics* 72:857–863, 1983.

Moore K: *Developing Human*, ed 2. Philadelphia, WB Saunders, 1977.

Moutsouris C: The "solid stage" and congenital intestinal atresia. *J Pediatr Surg* 1:446–450, 1966.

Muller F, Aubry M, Gasser B, Duchatel F, Boué J, Boué A: Prenatal diagnosis of cystic fibrosis. *Prenatal Diag* 5:109–117, 1985.

Muller F, O'Rahilly R: Cerebral dysraphia (future anencephaly) in a human twin embryo at stage 13. *Teratology* 30:167–177, 1984.

Munke M, Emanuel B, Zackai E: Holoprosencephaly: Association with interstitial deletion of 2p and review of the cytogenetic literature. *Am J Med Genet* 30:929–938, 1988.

Myrianthopoulos N, Melnick M: Studies in neural tube defects. I. *Am J Med Genet* 26:783–796, 1987.

Nishimura H, Okamoto N: Iniencephaly, in Vinken P, and Bruyn G (eds): *Congenital Malformations of the Brain and Skull. Handbook of Clinical Neurology*, vol 30, Amsterdam, Elsevier North Holland Publishing Co., 1977, p 257.

Nixon H, Tawes R: Etiology and treatment of small intestinal atresia. *Surgery* 69:41–51, 1971.

Nora J, Fraser C: *Medical Genetics. Principles and Practice*, ed 3. Philadelphia, Lea & Fabiger, 1989.

Nora J, Nora A: *Genetics and Conselling in Cardiovascular Diseases*. Springfield, IL, Charles C Thomas, 1978.

Norio R, Kaariainen H, Rapola J, Herva R, Kekomaki M: Familial congenital diaphragmatic defects. *Am J Med Genet* 17:471–483, 1984.

Ossipof V, Hall BD: Etiologic factors in the amniotic band syndrome. A study of 24 patients. *Birth Defects* XIII(3D)117–132, 1977.

Osuna A, Lindham SS: Four cases of omphalocele in two generations of the same family. *Clin Genet* 9:354–356, 1976.

Padget D: Neuroschisis and human embryonic maldevelopment. J Neuropath Exp Neur 29:192–215, 1970.

Pagon R, Smith D, Shephard T: Urethral obstruction malformation complex: A cause of abdominal muscle deficiency and the "prune-belly." *J Pediatr* 94:900–906, 1979.

Pagon RA, Stephens TD, McGillivray BC, Siebert JR, Wright VJ, Hsu LL, Poland BJ, Emanuel I, Hall JG: Body wall defects with reduction limb anomalies. A report of fifteen cases. March of Dimes Birth Defects Foundation. *Birth Defects* OAS 15(5A): 171–185, 1979.

Papp Z, Csecsei I, Toth Z, Polgar K, Szeifert G: Exencephaly in human fetuses. *Clin Genet* 30:440–444, 1986.

Patten B: Overgrowth of the neural tube in young human embryos. *Anat Rec* 113:381–393, 1952.

Patten B: Embryological stages in the establishing of myeloschisis with spina bifida. *Am J Anat* 93:365–395, 1953.

Pena S, Shokeir M: Syndrome of camptodactyly, multiple ankyloses, facial anomalies, and pulmonary hypoplasia: a lethal condition. *J Pediatr* 85:373–375, 1974.

Pinsky L: The syndromology of anorectal malformation (atresia, stenosis, ectopia). *Am J Med Genet* 1:461–474, 1978.

Pinsky L, Kaufman M: Genetics of steroid receptors and their disorders, in Harris H, Hirschorn K (eds): *Advances in Human Genetics*, 1987, pp 299–472.

Poland BJ, Miller JR, Harris M, Livingston J: Spontaneous abortion: A study of 1961 women and their conceptuses. *Acta Obstet Gynecol Scand* [Suppl] 102:5–32, 1981.

Potier M, Cousineau J, Michaud L, Zolinger M, Melancon S, Dallaire L: Fetal intestinal microvilli in human amniotic fluid. *Prenatal Diag* 6:429–436, 1986.

Potter E, Craig J: Pathology of the fetus and the infant. Chicago, Year Book Medical Publishers, 1975, p 303.

Powers J, Tummons R, Caviness V, Moser A, Moser H: Structural and chemical alterations in the cerebral maldevelopment of fetal cerebro-hepato-renal (Zellweger) syndrome. *J Neuropath Exp Neurol* 48:270–289, 1989.

Puri P, Gorman F: Lethal nonpulmonary anomalies associated with congenital diaphragmatic hernia: Implications for early uterine surgery. *J Pediatr Surg* 19:29–32, 1984.

Reeders S, Gal A, Propping P, Waldherr R, Davies K, Zerres K, Hogenkamp T, Schmidt W, Dolata M, Weatherall D: Prenatal diagnosis of autosomal dominant polycystic kidney disease with a DNA probe. *Lancet* ii:6–7, 1986.

Risdon R: The urogenital System, in Keeling JW (ed): *Fetal and Neonatal Pathology*. Berlin Heidelberg New York, Springer-Verlag, 1987, p 407.

Romero R, Pilu G, Jeanty P, Ghidini A, Hobbins J: *Prenatal Diagnosis of Congenital Anomalies*. Norwalk, CT, Appleton and Lange, 1988.

Roodhooft A, Birnholz J, Holmes L: Familial nature of congenital absence and severe dysgenesis of both kidneys. *New Engl J Med* 310:1341–1345, 1984.

Ross J, Frias J: Microcephaly, in Vinken P, and Bruyn G (eds): *Congenital Malformations of the Brain and Skull, Handbook of Clinical Neurology*, vol 30, Amsterdam, Elsevier North Holland Publishing Co, 1977.

Ryynanen M, Sepala M, Kuusela P, Rapola J, Aula P, Seppa A, Jokela V, Castren O: Antenatal screening for congenital nephrosis in Finland by maternal serum α-fetoprotein. *Br J Obstet Gynaecol* 90:437–442, 1983.

Saenger P: Abnormal sex differentiation. *J Pediatr* 104:1–14, 1984.

Salinas C, Bartoshesky L, Othersen H, Leape L, Feingold M, Jorgenson R: Familial occurrence of gastroschisis. *Am J Dis Child* 133:514–517, 1979.

Schubert-Staudacher E, Jauch H: Two sibs with bilateral diaphragmatic defect. *Clin Genet* 26:485–487, 1984.

Seed JW, Cefalo RC, Herbert WNP: Amniotic band syndrome. *Am J Obstet Gynecol* 144:243–248, 1982.

Seller M: Periconceptional vitamin supplementation to prevent recurrence of neural tube defects. *Lancet* ii:1392–1393, 1985.

Seller M, Kalousek D: Neural tube defects: Heterogeneity and homogeneity. *Am J Med Genet* [Suppl] 2:77–87, 1986.

Seller M, Creasy M, Aberman E: Alphafetoprotein levels in amniotic fluids from spontaneous abortions. *Br Med J* 1:1600, 1974.

Sheppard S, Nevin N, Seller M, Wild J, Smithells R, Read A, Harris R, Fielding D, Schorah C: Neural tube defect recurrence after 'partial' vitamin supplementation. J Med Genet 26:326–329, 1989.

Simpson J: *Disorders of Sexual Differentiation*. New York, Academic Press, 1976.

Simpson J: Disorders of gonads and internal reproductive ducts, in Emery, Rimoin (eds): *Principles and Practice of Medical Genetics*, vol 2. Edinburgh, Churchill Livingston, 1983, p 1227.

Smith D: *Recognizable Patterns of Human Malformation*. Philadelphia, WB Saunders, 1982, p 472.

Smith D, Bartlett C, Harrah L: Monozygotic twinning and the Duhamel anomalad (imperforate anus to sirenomelia): A nonrandom association between two aberrations in morphogenesis. *Birth Defects* OAS XII:53–63, 1976.

Smith E: The early development of the trachea and esophagus in relation to atresia of the esophagus and tracheo-esophageal fistula. Carnegie Institute of Washington, Pub 611. *Contributions to embryology* 36:41–57, 1957.

Spranger J, Langer L, Wiedemann H: *Bone Dysplasias: An Atlas of Constitutional Disorders of Skeletal Development*. Philadelphia, WB Saunders, 1974.

Stocker J, Madewell J, Drake R: Congenital cystic adenomatoid malformation of the lung. *Hum Pathol* 8:155–171, 1977.

Swinyard C, Chaube S, Nishimura H: Embryogenetic aspects of human meningomyelocele. *Pediatr Ann* 2:26–43, 1973.

Tanimura T: Complete dysraphism in human embryos. *Teratology* 8:107, 1973.

Temtamy S, McKusick V: *The Genetics of Hand Malformations*. New York, Alan R. Liss, Inc., 1978.

Thorburn M, Wright E, Miller C, Smith-Read E: Exomphalosmacroglossia-gigantism syndrome in Jamaican infants. *Am J Dis Child* 119:316–321, 1970.

Tokunaka S, Koyanagi T, Tsuji I: Two infantile cases of primary megalo-ureter with uncommon pathological findings: Ultrastructural study and its clinical implication. *J Urol* 123:214, 1980a.

Tokunaka S, Koyanagi T, Matsuno T, Gotoh T, Tsuji I: Paraureteral diverticula: Clinical experience with 17 cases associated with renal dysmorphism. *J Urol* 124:791, 1980b.

Toriello H, Higgins J: Possible causal heterogeneity in spina bifida cystica. *Am J Med Genet* 21:13–20, 1985.

Torpin R: *Fetal Malformations Caused by Amnion Rupture During Gestation.* Springfield, IL, Charles C Thomas, 1968.

Toyama W: Combined congenital defects of the anterior abdominal wall, sternum, diaphragm, pericardium and heart: A case report and review of the syndrome. *Pediatrics* 50:778–792, 1972.

Van Allen MI, Curry C, Gallagher L: Limb body wall complex: I. Pathogenesis. *Am J Med Genet* 28:529–548, 1987a.

Van Allen MI, Curry C, Walden C, Gallagher L, Patten R: Limb-body wall complex: II. Limb and spine defects. *Am J Med Genet* 28:549–565, 1987b.

van der Putte SCJ, Van Limborgh J: The embryonic development of the main lymphatics in man. *Acta Morphol Neerl-Scand* 18:323–335, 1980.

van der Rest M, Hayes A, Maric P, Desbarats M, Kaplan P, Glorieux FH: Lethal osteogenesis imperfecta with amniotic band lesions. Collagen studies. *Am J Med Genet* 24:433–446, 1986.

Van Praagh R: The segmental approach to diagnosis in congenital heart disease. *Birth Defects* 8:4–23, 1972.

Van Staey M, De Bie S, Matton T, De Roose J: Familial congenital esophageal atresia. *Hum Genet* 66:260–266, 1984.

Vorherr H: Factors influencing fetal growth. *Am J Obstet Gynecol* 142:577–588, 1982.

Warkany J: *Congenital Malformations.* Chicago, Year Book Medical Publishers, 1971.

Warkany J, Lemire R, Cohen M: *Mental Retardation and Congenital Malformations of the Central Nervous System.* Chicago, Year Book Medical Publishers, 1981.

Warshaw J: Perspectives on intrauterine growth retardation. *Growth Genet Horm* 2:1–6, 1986.

Wells L: Development of the human diaphragm and pleural sac. Carnegie Contributions to Embryology No. 236, 35:107–134, 1954.

Wigger H, Blanc W: The prune belly syndrome, in Sommers S, Rosen P (eds): *Pathology Annual.* Part I vol 12. New York, Appleton-Century Crofts, 1977, p 17.

Wigglesworth J, Desai R, Guerrini P: Fetal lung hypoplasia: Biochemical and structural variations and their possible significance. *Arch Dis Child* 56:606–615, 1981.

Wilson R, Baird P: Renal agenesis in British Columbia. *Am J Med Genet* 21:153–165, 1985.

Wolff G: Familial congenital diaphragmatic defect: Review and conclusions. *Hum Genet* 54:1–5, 1980.

Wolter J, Kroblich R, Ravin J: Synophthalmus and anencephaly. *J Pediatr Ophthal* 5:217–223, 1968.

Young ID, Lindenbaum RH, Thompson EM, Pemburg ME: Amniotic bands in connective tissue disorders. *Arch Dis Child* 60:1061–1063, 1985.

hybridization (Cradock-Watson et al., 1989). Therapeutic abortions carried out because of acquisition of or contact with rubella in pregnancy are frequent. In Great Britain, Miller et al. (1982) reported that 94% mothers who acquired rubella in the first trimester underwent therapeutic abortion.

Herpes Group Viruses

The herpes group of viruses includes cytomegalovirus (CMV), herpes simplex virus (HSV), varicella zoster virus (VZV), and Epstein-Barr virus (EBV). The complexity of this group makes it difficult to evaluate fetal infection since it may be due to primary maternal infection or to the reactivation of an old infection during pregnancy. As a general rule, primary maternal herpes virus infection during pregnancy is more likely to cause fetal morbidity or mortality. Of this group, CMV is most commonly associated with intrauterine infection. The manifestations of fetal CMV infection include intrauterine growth retardation, hepatosplenomegaly, hepatitis with hyperbilirubinemia, pneumonitis, encephalitis, cerebral calcification, and microcephaly (Peckman and Marshall, 1983).

The majority of HSV fetal infections are caused by HSV Type 2 following rupture of membranes or during passage of the fetus through an infected birth canal. Rarely, the fetus may become infected following a primary maternal infection during pregnancy. Developmental defects include microcephaly, intracranial calcifications, chorioretinitis, and microphthalmia (Hanshaw et al., 1985).

Approximately 95% of women of child-bearing age have serologic evidence of past varicella-zoster virus (Herpesvirus varicellae) infection. Although congenital varicella and pattern of anomalies associated with it are recognized, primary varicella infection in pregnancy and fetal loss are rare.

There are no convincing reports of EBV infection associated with fetal loss in the literature.

Influenza

A causal relationship between influenza and developmental defects remains unclear (Leck, 1963). High fetal loss, however, was reported in the influenza pandemic of 1918–1920, especially when the disease was complicated by pneumonia (Holzel, 1987).

Enteroviruses

These include Coxsackie viruses A and B, ECHO virus, poliovirus, and all of the picornavirus group. None of these viruses have been positively associated with an increase in develomental defects. Spontaneous abortion has been observed following documented Coxsackie A16 infection and poliovirus infection in the first trimester, but causal association has not been established (Ogilvie and Tearne, 1980; Siegal and Greenberg, 1956).

Hepatitis A and B Viruses

No increase in fetal loss or in the frequency of developmental defects has been reported after either hepatitis A (HAV) or hepatitis B (HBV) maternal infection. Claims of an association between HAV infection and trisomy 21 syndrome (Stoller and Collman, 1965) have not been supported (Kucera, 1970). After primary infection with HBV during the first or second trimester, transmission to the fetus is unlikely. In third trimester maternal infection with HBV, 60 to 70% of infants are infected, since the virus is most commonly transmitted at delivery (Schweitzer et al., 1973).

Parvovirus

Spontaneous abortion of fetuses that may be hydropic is reported to occur after parvovirus B19 infection. The hydrops fetalis seen in this infection is the result of anemia due to red blood cell destruction. Histologic features consist of excessive iron pigment in the liver, hepatitis, a leukoerythroblastic reaction, and eosinophilic changes in hematopoietic cell nuclei (Anand et al., 1987). In situ hybridization with radiolabeled viral DNA has been used to confirm the diagnosis.

Fig. VII-1. (a) 17½-week male fetus terminated for suspected rubella infection due to maternal exposure. Note the appropriate development and the lack of any developmental defect. No evidence of fetal infection was detected on culture. (b) Products of pregnancy termination (D&E) for suspected rubella infection. Both the fetus (16 weeks of development) and the placenta are fragmented; arrows, fetal skull and chest. The placenta tested positive for rubella virus, but the fetal organs tested negative.

Fig. VII-2. (a) A 16-week female fetus with a cytomegalovirus infection, showing severe intrauterine growth retardation, ascites, and markedly enlarged placenta. (b) Enlarged liver, with necrosis and calcifications (arrows) from the same fetus.

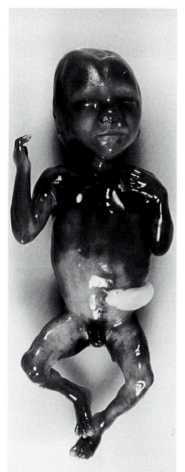

VII-1a

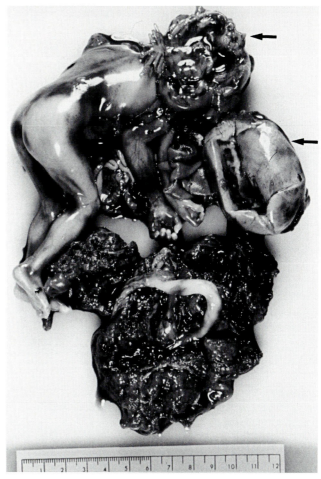

VII-1b

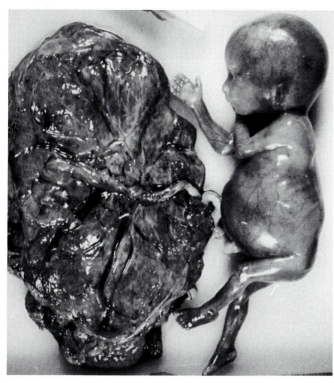

VII-2a

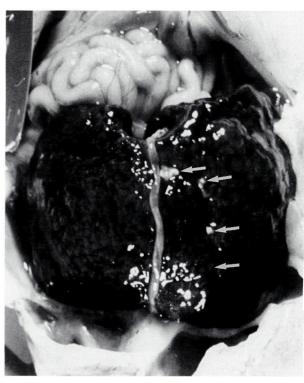

VII-2b

Human Immunodeficiency Virus

Congenital human immunodeficiency virus (HIV) infections (AIDS) have been reported and an estimate of in utero transmission is in the range of 50 to 65%. Transplacental transmission is indicated by either positive virus cultures from aborted 14- to 20-week fetuses or from cord blood (Sprecher et al., 1986). The exact pathway of transmission remains unknown, but transplacental passage by a cell-associated virus is likely (Jauniaux et al., 1988). There are no well-documented cases of HIV infection causing specific dysmorphic features or malformations (Feinkind and Minkoff, 1988).

Bacterial Infections

Bacterial infections in the fetus are more frequently recognized than viral, parasitic, or fungal infections. In most cases, acquisition of the organism is from the maternal genital tract via an ascending route. Premature rupture of membranes or a sudden spontaneous abortion, may be the first indication of intrauterine infection. Although ascending infection from the maternal genital tract is probably the most common route, there are a number of other possibilities, including (1) direct infection from the maternal peritoneal cavity, (2) iatrogenic infection during such prenatal procedures as amniocentesis, and (3) hematogenous maternal infection. In addition, bacteria can be carried asymptomatically in the male urogenital tract (Taylor-Robinson, 1987). An association between coitus, chorioamnionitis, and premature rupture of membranes has been suggested (Naeye, 1982). It was reported by Hameed et al. (1984) that intact membranes do not prevent bacteria from gaining access to the amniotic fluid.

Infection during a previable second trimester pregnancy caused by bacteria usually leads to pregnancy loss. The most frequent organisms associated with ascending intrauterine infection are listed in Table VII-1. The typical manifestation of bacterial infection is inflammation of the placental membranes and the chorionic plate, decidua, and umbilical cord. This inflammatory process is termed *chorioamnionitis* because the first signs of inflammation are usually found beneath the amnion and along the surface of the chorion.

Whether the infection occurs prior to rupture of the membranes by invasion of the amniotic sac through devitalized

TABLE VII.1. Bacterial pathogens associated with chorioamnionitis.

Gram-positive bacteria	Gram-negative bacteria	Other bacteria
Group B streptococci	*Bacteroides* sp.	*Ureaplasma urealyticum*
Listeria monocytogenes	Coliform bacteria	*Chlamydia* sp.
Coagulate-negative staphylococci	*Hemophilus* sp.	*Mycoplasma hominis*
Viridans streptococci	*Brucella* sp.	*Treponema pallidum*
Group D streptococci	*Neisseria gonorrhoeae*	*Borrelia* sp.
Anaerobic Gram-positive cocci	*Campylobacter* sp.	*Mobiluncus* sp.
Lactobacilli	*Fusobacterium* sp.	*Gardnerella vaginalis*
	Miscellaneous nonfermentative bacteria (*Pseudomonas; Aeromonas*)	

membranes over the uterine os, or is secondary to it, is not clear. Once bacteria are in the amniotic sac, they cause maternal leukocyte migration from the intervillous space toward the amniotic cavity. This leads to a gross loss of translucency of the membrane, which becomes creamy yellow. Most bacteria infect the membranes diffusely. Inhalation and ingestion of infected amniotic fluid by the fetus (*amniotic infection syndrome*) can be diagnosed microscopically by sectioning the fetal lungs and stomach. When infection spreads to the fetus in this manner, it can cause intrauterine aspiration pneumonia (Chapter VI) or develop into septicemia. Intrauterine death may occur prior to spontaneous abortion when the infecting agent is strongly virulent, as is the case with group B streptococci.

Acute chorioamnionitis frequently induces labor, presumably because the neutrophils and bacteria that are present release phospholipases, which, in turn, enzymatically release arachidonic acid from the fetal membranes (Romero et al., 1986). The arachidonic acid rapidly converts to prostaglandin E_2 and to F_2a. Prostaglandin E_2 causes the cervix to dilate and F_2a initiates uterine contractions.

In many cases, the infection extends into the decidua basalis, from which bacteria may reach the fetus by being

Fig. VII-3. Acute chorioamnionitis in a fresh fetus of 20 developmental weeks. Note the milky appearance of the fetal vessels on the chorionic surface (arrows).

Fig. VII-4. Severe chorioamnionitis and a fresh fetus of 17 developmental weeks. Note the diffuse discoloration of the fetal surface.

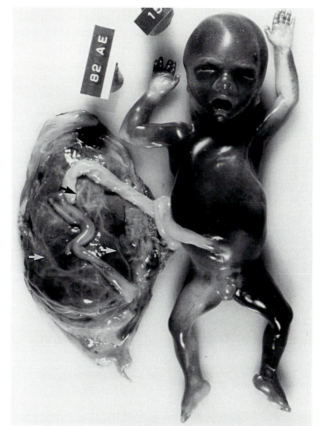

VII-3

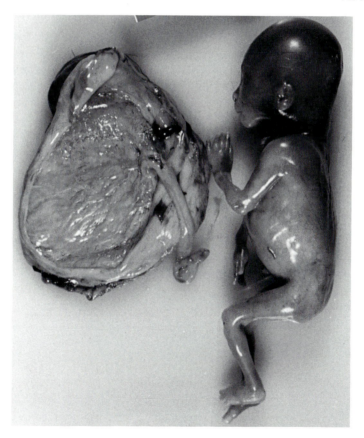

VII-4

shed into the intervillous blood (Cooperman et al., 1980). The villi appear to form an effective barrier to the transfer of most bacteria but do not seem to hinder passage of *Listeria monocytogenes* and *Treponema pallidum*. Hematogenously acquired infections are less commonly associated with pregnancy loss and/or intrauterine fetal death than ascending infections. *Listeria* causes a necrotizing villitis and chorioamnionitis in placenta. The fetus shows numerous granulomata in all internal viscera. Syphilis of the fetus and placenta generally occurs late in pregnancy and is not observed among previable fetuses.

Infections with Other Microorganisms

Fungi

Despite the frequency and ease with which fungi, specifically *Candida* sp., are isolated from genital tracts of pregnant patients, antenatal fetal fungal infections are rare. Discrete rounded yellow plaques, varying in size from 0.5 to 2 mm, seen in the umbilical cord and membranes represent pathognomonic changes. As the organisms penetrate the surface epithelium of the cord and amnion, they evoke a very dense cellular response by polymorphonuclear and mononuclear cells. Evidence of inflammatory changes affecting the chorionic villi or decidual plate is not usually found (Whyte et al., 1982).

Mycoplasma and *Chlamydia*

The role of mycoplasma in spontaneous abortion is unclear. Genital mycoplasmas, *Mycoplasma hominis* and *Ureaplasma urealyticum*, were implicated in the etiology of repeated spontaneous abortion when it was shown that the organisms were isolated more often from the cervix and the endometrium of habitual aborters than from those of controls (Naesseus et al., 1987; Quinn et al., 1987).

The isolation of genital mycoplasmas in conceptuses spontaneously lost prior to 20 weeks of gestation has been described (Freiberg, 1980), and colonization of endometrium,

placental membranes, and amniotic fluid by genital mycoplasmas has been demonstrated at amniocentesis in the second trimester (Cassel et al., 1983). Amniotic fluids collected from patients with clinical intramniotic infection also show a high incidence of *Mycoplasma hominis* (Blanco et al., 1983).

Mycoplasma hominis and *U. urealyticum* have been isolated with greater frequency from couples with pregnancy losses than from couples with successful outcome, and detailed serologic investigation suggest that certain *Ureaplasma* serotypes may be more pathogenic than others (Quinn et al., 1987).

Colonization of the female genital tract by *Chlamydia trachomatis* is commonly described, but no significant evidence of *Chlamydia* involvement in the early pregnancy loss has been reported (Schachter, 1978). *Chlamydia trachomatis* infections have been reported in a few premature infants and stillbirths but not in previable fetuses (Martin et al., 1982).

Toxoplasma gondii

Infection with the parasite *T. gondii* follows an exposure to the oocysts in cat excreta or infected soil, or the consumption of contaminated meats. Most maternal infections are asymptomatic or result in a mild, influenza-like illness. Infection in early pregnancy may induce an abortion. Recurrent spontaneous abortion caused by chronic toxoplasmosis has been reported by Remington (1973), who found that although abortion in chronically infected women may occur, it is not frequent. The frequency of fetal infection is increased in the later stages of pregnancy. Maternal infection in the third trimester results in 59% affected fetuses, whereas only 14% are affected after first trimester and 29% after second trimester infections (Desmonts and Couvreur, 1979). Fetal manifestations include intrauterine growth retardation, hepatomegaly, meningoencephalitis, hydrocephalus, intracranial calcifications, and chorioretinitis.

Malaria

Prenatally acquired malaria is more common among fetuses of nonimmune mothers who contract malaria during preg-

Fig. VII-5. Severe chorioamnionitis in a retained macerated fetus of 9½ developmental weeks. Note the discoloration of the fetal surface.

Fig. VII-6. A 16½-week fetus, showing a collection of pus under the pleura of the right lung. Cultures grew *Listeria monocytogenes*.

Fig. VII-7. A 16½-week, female fetus with no developmental abnormalities; the placenta shows a mild opaqueness of the fetal surface. Both the fetal lungs and the stomach and placenta tested positive for *Mycoplasma*.

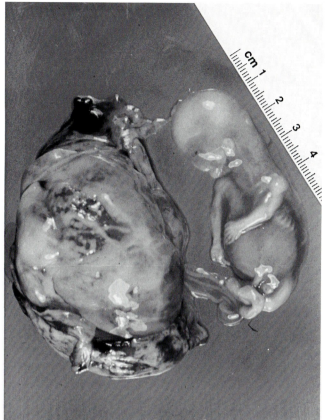

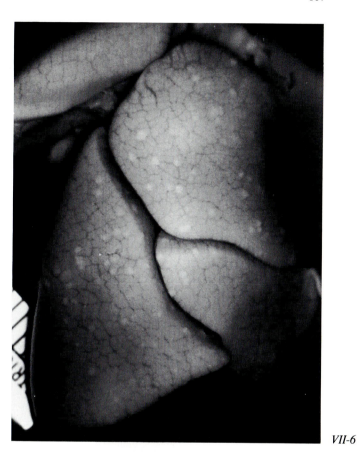

VII-5   *VII-6*

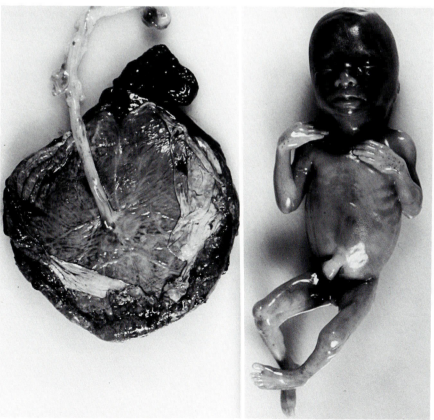

VII-7

nancy than among the indigenous population of malarial areas, in spite of the regular infestation of the placenta in these cases (Ransome-Kuti, 1972). The incidence of abortion has also been shown to be inversely proportional to the degrees of maternal immunity.

References

Anand A, Gray E, Brown T, Clewley PJ, Cohen BJ: Human parvovirus infection in pregnancy and hydrops fetalis. *New Engl J Med* 316:183–186, 1987.

Blanco JD, Gibbs RS, Malherbe H, Strickland-Cholmley M, St. Clair PJ, Castaneda YS: A controlled study of genital mycoplasmas in amniotic fluid from patients with intra-amniotic infection. *J Infect Dis* 147:650–653, 1983.

Boué A, Loffredo V: Avortment cause par le virus dl'herpes type II. Isolement du virus à partir de cultures de tissues zygotiques. *Presse Med* 78:103–106, 1970.

Cassell GM, Davis OR, Waites KB, Brown MB, Marriott PA, Stagus S, Davis JK: Isolation of *Mycoplasma hominis* and *Ureaplasma urealyticum* from amniotic fluid at 16–20 weeks of gestation. *Sex Trans Dis* 10:294–302, 1983.

Cooperman NR, Kasin M, Rajaschekazaiah KR: Clinical significance of amniotic fluid, amniotic membranes and endometrial biopsy cultures at the time of caesarean section. *Am J Obstet Gynecol* 137:936–941, 1980.

Cradock-Watson JE, Miller E, Ridehalgh MKS, Terry GM, Ho-Terry L: Detection of rubella virus in fetal and placental tissues and in the throats of neonates after serologically confirmed rubella in pregnancy. *Prenat Diag* 9:91–96, 1989.

Desmonts G, Couvreur J: Congenital toxoplasmosis: A prospective study of the offspring of 542 women who acquired toxoplasmosis during pregnancy. Pathophysiology of congenital disease, in Thalhammer O, Baumgarten K, Pollack A (eds): *Proceedings of the Sixth European Congress on Perinatal Medicine, Vienna.* Stuttgart, Thieme, 1979, pp 51–60.

Feinkind L, Minkoff HL: HIV in pregnancy. *Clin Perinatol* 15:189–202, 1988.

Freiberg J: Mycoplasmas and ureaplasmas in infertility and abortion. *Fertil Steril* 33:351–359, 1980.

Hameed S, Tejani N, Verma VL, Archibald F: Silent chorioamnionitis as a cause of preterm labour refractory to tocolytic therapy. *Am J Obstet Gynecol* 149:726, 1984.

Hanshaw JB, Dudgeon JA, Marshall WC (eds): Herpes simplex infection of the fetus and newborn, in *Viral Diseases of the Fetus and Newborn,* ed 2. Philadelphia, WB Saunders, 1985, vol 17, pp 132–153.

Holzel M: Infection in pregnancy and the neonatal period, in Keeling JW (ed): *Fetal and Neonatal Pathology.* Berlin Heidelberg New York, Springer-Verlag, 1987, pp 265–293.

Jauniaux E, Nessmann C, Imbert MC, Meuris S, Puissant F, Hustin J: Morphological aspects of the placenta in HIV pregnancies. *Placenta* 9:633–642, 1988.

Kucera J: Down's syndrome and infectious hepatitis. *Lancet* i:569–570, 1970.

Leck I: Incidence of malformations following influenza epidemics. *Br J Prev Soc Med* 17:70–80, 1963.

Martin DM, Koutsky L, Eschenbach DA, Daling RJ, Alexander RE, Benedetti JK, Holmes KK: Prematurity and perinatal mortality in pregnancies complicated by maternal *Chlamydia trachomatis* infections. *JAMA* 247:1585–1588, 1982.

Miller E, Cradock-Watson JE, Pollock TM: Consequences of confirmed maternal rubella at successive stages of pregnancy. *Lancet* ii:781–784, 1982.

Naesseus A, Foulan W, Cammu H, Goossens A, Lauwers S: Epidemiology and pathogenesis of *Ureaplasma urealyticum* in spontaneous abortion and early preterm labor. *Acta Obstet Gynecol Scand* 66:513–516, 1987.

Naeye RL: Factors that predispose to premature rupture of the fetal membranes. *Obstet Gynecol* 60:93–97, 1982.

Ogilvie MM, Tearne FC: Spontaneous abortion after hand- foot- and mouth disease caused by Coxsackie virus A16. *Br Med J* 281:1527–1528, 1980.

Peckham C, Marshall WC: Infections in pregnancy, in Barron SL, Thompson AM (eds): *Obstetric Epidemiology.* London, Academic Press, 1983, pp 209–262.

Quinn PA, Butany J, Taylor J, Hannah W: Chorioamnionitis: Its association with pregnancy outcome and microbial infection. *Am J Obstet Gynecol* 156:379–387, 1987.

Ransome-Kuti O: Malaria in childhood. *Paediatrics* 19:319–340, 1972.

Remington JS: Toxoplasmosis, in Charles D, Finlaid L (eds): *Obstetric and Perinatal Infections.* Philadelphia, Lea and Febiger, 1973, p 27.

Romero R, Emamian M, Quintero R, Wan H, Hobbins JC, Mitchell MD: Amniotic fluid prostaglandin levels and intra amniotic infections. *Lancet* i:1380, 1986.

Schachter J: Chlamydial infections. *N Engl J Med* 298:490–495, 1978.

Schweitzer IL, Moseley JW, Aschcavai M, et al.: Factors influencing neonatal infection by hepatitis B virus. *Gastroenterology* 65:277–283, 1973.

Siegal M, Greenberg M: Poliomyelitis in pregnancy: Effect on fetus and newborn infant. *J Pediatr* 49:280–288, 1956.

Sprecher S, Soumenkoff G, Puissant F, Degueldre M: Vertical transmission of HIV in 15-week fetus. *Lancet* ii:288–289, 1986.

Stoller A, Collman RD: Evidence of infective hepatitis followed by Down's syndrome nine months later. *Lancet* ii:1221–1223, 1965.

Taylor-Robinson: The male reservoir of *Ureaplasma urealyticum.* *Paed Infect Dis* 6 (Suppl 5):S234, 1987.

Thorp JM, Jr, Katz VL, Fowler LJ, Kurtzman JT, Bowes WA, Jr: Fetal death from chlamydial infection across intact amniotic membranes. *Am J Obstet Gynecol* 161:1245–1246, 1989.

Whyte RK, Hussain Z, deSa D: Antenatal infections with *Candida* species. *Arch Dis Child* 57:528–535, 1982.

CHAPTER VIII

Chromosomal Abnormalities and Embryonic Phenotype

Introduction

Pregnancy loss during the embryonic period of development is a common event. Among the estimated 15 to 20% of clinically recognized pregnancies that are lost, the majority take place when the conceptus is undergoing embryonic development. The abnormal morphology of aborted embryos has been noted by earlier authors (Mall, 1908; Hertig et al., 1936). It has since been recognized that the incidence of cytogenetic abnormalities among such embryonic spontaneous abortions is over 50% (Boué et al., 1975; Jacobs and Hassold, 1987), with chromosomal trisomy, monosomy, and polyploidy being the most common. Nearly all these chromosomal defects are "de novo," arising either during parental gametogenesis or fertilization/cleavage. Trisomies and monosomies are caused by meiotic chromosomal nondisjunction; triploidy usually results from double fertilization of an ova by two sperms and tetraploidy from abnormal cleavage. Many studies have been dedicated to answering the question whether an abortion with an identified chromosomal defect—specifically, chromosomal trisomy—predisposes the parents to the higher risk of having a liveborn infant with chromosomal trisomy. When allowance was made for maternal age, no association between spontaneous abortion with aneuploidy and an increased risk of a future liveborn infant with a chromosomal defect could be demonstrated (Warburton et al., 1987).

No specific embryonic or placental phenotypes correspond to the various chromosomal defects seen during the embryonic period. The embryonic phenotype can vary from completely normal, as seen occasionally in chromosomal triploidy, to complete disorganization of embryonic growth. The same variability is seen in the development of the gestational sac and the chorionic villi. Only in triploidy do the villous changes appear to be specific (see below), in most cases. Claims that placental morphology correlates closely with

chromosomal complement (Honoré et al., 1976) have not been confirmed.

It is difficult to justify routine karyotyping of every early pregnancy loss. However, in specific cases, such as repeated pregnancy loss, or a history of infertility, it will help if the obstetrician knows the chromosomal complement of the conceptus. The presence of chromosomal trisomy does not indicate an increased chance of another aneuploid spontaneous abortion (Warburton et al., 1987). Triploidy, or tetraploidy, usually represents an accident of fertilization or cleavage, with no increased risk of repetition. If the chromosomal complement is normal, maternal hormonal insufficiency, uterine defects preventing a normal implantation, or a lethal genetic mutation should be suspected.

Trisomies

Trisomies represent the commonest chromosomal defect in early spontaneous abortuses. Trisomy for all chromosomes except chromosome number 1 has been described (Jacobs and Hassold, 1987). The frequency of various trisomies varies greatly. Trisomy 16 is found in 31% of trisomic conceptuses. The frequency of trisomies 2, 7, 13 to 15, 18, and 21 to 22 varies from 4 to 10%. Trisomies 4, 8, 9, 10, and 20 occur with a frequency of around 2 to 4%. The remaining trisomies are usually categorized as rare, with a frequency of 0.2 to 1% (Table VIII-1).

The morphology of trisomic conceptions is not predictable, although embryonic growth disorganization is the most common finding. It has been postulated that the *rare trisomies* always present as small, intact sacs with no embryo, which represents the most severe degree of growth disorganization (GD$_1$). However, even among rare trisomies, other pheno-

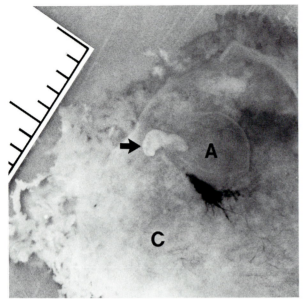

VIII-1a

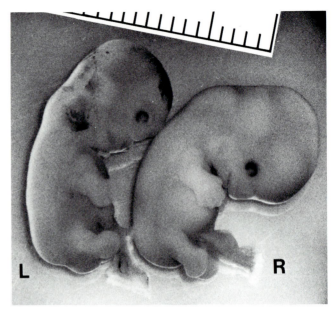

VIII-1b

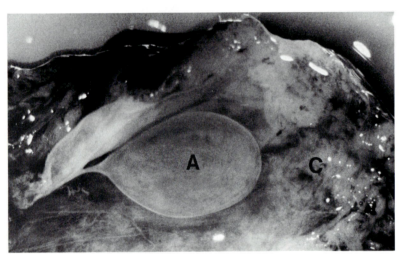

VIII-1c

Fig. VIII-1. Variable phenotypes of rare trisomies: (a) a trisomy 4 embryo (47,XY,+4), 2.5 mm in length with an midembryonic constriction due to aberrant amnion development. The neural tube is closed. The tail is short. A, amniotic sac; C, chorion; Arrow, an embryonic head. (b) A trisomy 5 embryo (Stage 18), left (L), is compared to a normal embryo (Stage 18), right (R). Note in the trisomic embryo the small head, cleft lip, and the slightly delayed development of both upper and lower limbs. The discoloration of trisomic embryo is due to maceration. (c) A focal trisomy 17 anembryonic sac (GD$_1$) with an intact amniotic sac (A) and an abundant chorionic villi (C).

Fig. VIII-2. Phenotypes of trisomies 13 and 14: (a) A trisomy 13 embryo, 15 mm in length, with a small head and a dysplastic facial area. A subectodermal hemorrhage is seen in the frontoparietal area. There is delayed development of the limb buds and shortening of the tail. The umbilical cord shows a cyst (C). (b) A trisomy 13, female, degenerated and damaged embryo (Stage 22). The major malformation consists of partial cyclopia, the proboscis (arrow) is above the fused orbits; there is also a postaxial polydactyly on the right hand and a common truncus in the heart (arrow). (c) A trisomy 13, incomplete embryo with microcephaly, bilateral cleft lip, and hyperpigmentation of eyes. (d) A trisomy 14 female embryo (Stage 18) with a large frontoparietal encephalocele (E) and facial dysplasia. (e) A trisomy 13 (Stage 16) degenerated embryo, with a body stalk and yolk sac, showing a defect of the caudal neural tube closure with an overgrowth of neural tissue (arrow).

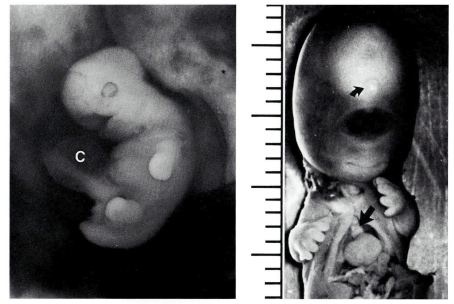

VIII-2a

VIII-2b

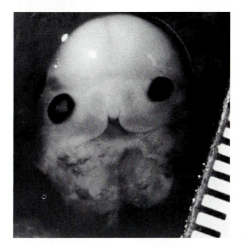

VIII-2c

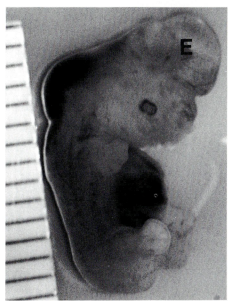

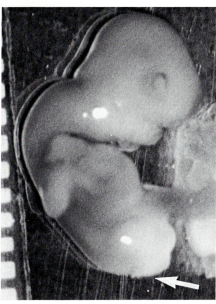

VIII-2d

VIII-2e

TABLE VIII.1. Frequency of chromosomal trisomies for individual chromosomes in spontaneous abortions.

Chromosome	Cases	Percent
1	0	0
2	32	4.9
3	6	0.9
4	15	2.3
5	1	0.2
6	3	0.5
7	28	4.3
8	23	3.5
9	23	3.5
10	13	2.0
11	1	0.2
12	4	0.6
13	33	5.0
14	27	4.0
15	50	7.6
16	204	31.0
17	3	0.5
18	38	5.8
19	1	0.2
20	16	2.4
21	58	8.8
22	66	10.1
X	11	1.7

[a]Modified from Warburton et al., 1980.

types, such as GD$_2$, GD$_3$, GD$_4$ and advanced embryos with focal defects, are seen. Histologic findings in the chorionic sac correlate with the gross morphology. Empty sacs usually show sparse villi with hydropic stroma and a hypoplastic trophoblast. When a fresh embryo is present, villi are usually more abundant, their stroma is vascularized, and the villous vessels contain nucleated red blood cells. The retained macerated embryo typically is associated with fibrotic villi and collapsed vessels that, histologically, show embryonic red blood cells with or without signs of hemolysis.

Common trisomies involve chromosomes 2, 7, 13 to 15, 16, 18, and 21 to 22. Although any phenotype can occur, the most frequent is growth disorganization with a nodular or cylindrical embryo. Conceptions with trisomy 2 characteristically show an empty intact sac. In the case of trisomies 13 to 15, the embryos are usually developed beyond Stage 18 (week 6–7) and show such localized defects as microcephaly, cleft lip, and polydactyly. Microcephaly and facial clefting is a typical feature of the trisomies 13, 14, and 15. Polydactyly is more specific for trisomy 13. Neural tube defects, holoprosencephaly, and heart defects are also seen in trisomies 13–15.

The typical trisomy 16 phenotype consists of a nodular or cylindrical embryo. However, an empty sac or embryo with a focal defect such as neural tube defect does not exclude trisomy 16.

It is important to realize that although trisomy 21 is compatible with complete intrauterine development, less than 30% of trisomy 21 conceptions do survive. They usually spontaneously abort early, with the morphology varying from an empty, intact sac to a morphologically normal embryo.

Trisomy 18 conceptuses show morphologic variations similar to those seen in trisomy 21.

Trisomy 22 is a more common finding in spontaneous abortion than is trisomy 21. Most conceptuses abort as growth-disorganized embryos or embryos with localized defects.

There are no characteristic features of villus morphology in common trisomies, but the above-described correlation of their gross morphology with histologic findings applies.

Fig. VIII-3. A trisomy 22 abnormal embryo (47,XX,+22) with a small head, facial dysplasia, and marked delayed development of both the upper and lower limb buds. There is also a short cystic umbilical cord (C).

Fig. VIII-4. A trisomy 7, well-preserved embryo (Stage 12). External development is normal, except for ill-defined branchial arches; arrow, cranial end of the embryo.

Fig. VIII-5. A trisomy 18 abnormal embryo. The external abnormalities include microcephaly, with absent cervical flexion; dysplastic facial features, with a proboscis above the level of the eyes (arrow); delayed development of all the limb buds (UL and LL); and a 1-mm epidermal cyst in the upper chest area; C, umbilical cord.

Fig. VIII-6. Common phenotype of trisomy 16: (a) A nodular embryo (arrow), less than 1 mm in length, attached to the amniotic membrane. (b) A cylindrical embryo, 4 mm in length, attached to the amniotic membrane; arrow, retinal pigment.

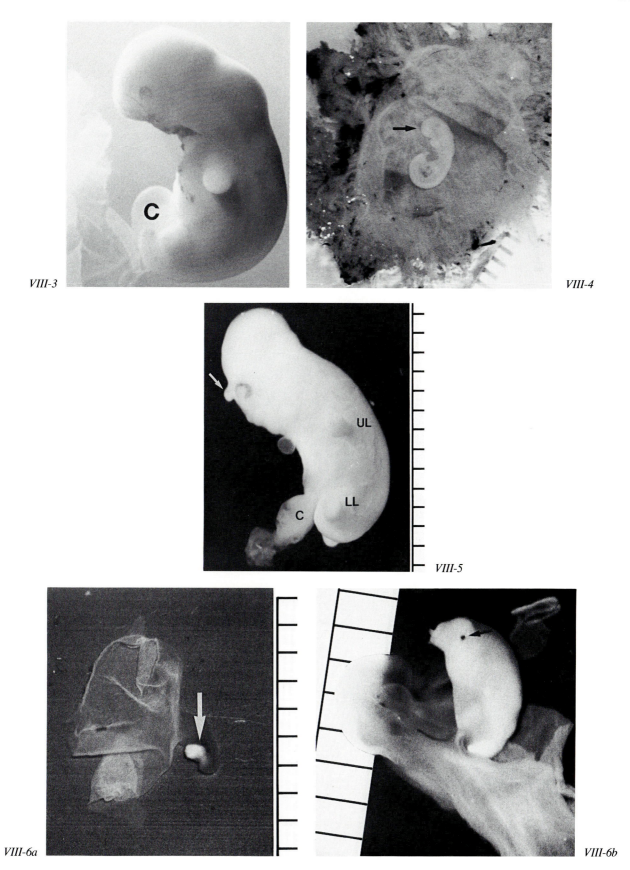

VIII-3

VIII-4

VIII-5

VIII-6a

VIII-6b

Monosomy X

It is interesting to note that, in spite of its high intrauterine lethality, the phenotype of monosomy X commonly involves normal or near-normal embryonic development (Table VIII-2). The 45,X embryos with focal defects are usually characterized by abnormal neural tube development in the form of cranial encephaloceles. Retarded development of the upper and lower limbs represents another feature of 45,X embryos with otherwise normal development. Most 45,X embryos are degenerated, due to their long intrauterine retention after intrauterine death. The embryonic phenotype never resembles the fetal phenotype, which is characterized by a posterior cervical hygroma and generalized subcutaneous edema.

The Breus mole commonly described in 45,X abortuses represents a recent subchorionic hemorrhage in a retained gestational sac.

TABLE VIII.2. Correlation of morphology and karyotype in 256 complete early abortion specimens.[a]

Morphology	Normal karyotype	Trisomy[b]	Monosomy X	Triploidy	Tetraploidy	Structural rearrangement
GD$_1$	15	13	2	1	3	3
GD$_2$	6	12	–	2	1	–
GD$_3$	10	11	–	–	–	1
GD$_4$	5	2	1	–	–	–
Normal embryos	32	4	5	3	–	1
Embryos with localized defects	10	29	18	25	–	7
Fragmented/degenerated embryos	8	13	2	7	2	2
Total	86	84	28	38	6	14

[a]From Kalousek DK: Anatomic and chromosome anomalies in specimens of early spontaneous abortion: Seven-year experience. In Gilbert EF, Opitz JM (eds): "Genetic Aspects of Developmental Pathology." New York: Alan R. Liss, Inc. for the March of Dimes Birth Defects Foundation BD:OAS 23(1):153–168, 1987, with permission from the copyright holder.
[b]Includes double trisomy.

Fig. VIII-7. Phenotype of 45,X complement: (a) An abnormal embryo (45,X), 18 mm CR length. The external abnormalities include microcephaly, lack of cervical flexion, midfacial dysplasia (arrow), and delayed development of the limb buds. (b) A damaged, abnormal embryo (45,X), with a microcephalic head and an encephalocele in the parietal area. Both the upper and lower limbs show delayed development. (c) A severely damaged embryo (45,X), with an intact hand and feet (long arrows), developed to Stage 20. Note the misplaced eyes (short arrow).

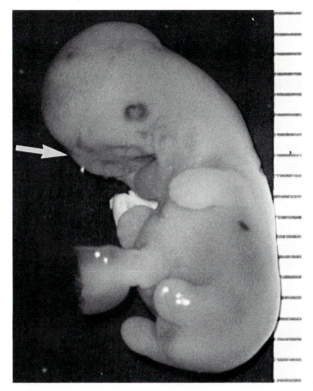

VIII-7a

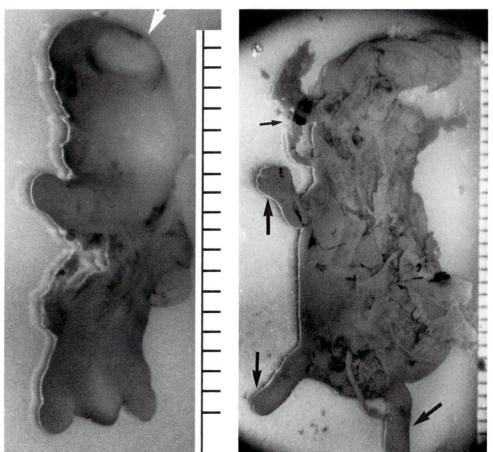

VIII-7b

VIII-7c

Triploidy

Triploidy is found in 17% of chromosomally abnormal spontaneous abortuses. Unlike tetraploidy, the majority of specimens show advanced embryonic development. Growth disorganization is rare (Table VIII-2). Although completely normal embryonic development is occasionally present, embryos with a typical abnormal phenotype are usually found. The features of this phenotype are as follows (Harris et al., 1981):

1. Limb retardation (upper and lower) relative to developmental age, established by CR length and retinal pigment development.
2. Facial dysplasia.
3. Symmetric or midline subectodermal hemorrhages.
4. Frequent neural tube defect in the lower spine.

Placental changes associated with triploidy in the embryonic stage of development are usually focal. Grossly the villi show cystic dilations. Histologically the changes consist of trophoblastic hyperplasia, usually moderate in degree and confined to the syncytial layer, and focal villus swelling with cistern formation. Cisterns are well-demarcated central fluid collections rimmed by mesenchyme of decreased vascularity and cellularity. Other histological features of early placental triploid tissue are scalloping of villous outlines and trophoblastic inclusions in the villous stroma (Szulman, 1987).

Fig. VIII-8. Phenotype of triploidy: (a) A degenerated embryo Stage 17 (69,XXX). The embryo is damaged at the lower face, neck, and upper thoracic area. Except for the shortening of the tail, no developmental abnormalities are identified. Two cysts lined by amnion are attached to the umbilical cord (arrows). (b) An abnormal embryo, 12-mm CRL (69,XXY). The embryo is damaged at the lower face, neck, and upper chest. It shows microcephaly, severe growth retardation of all the limb buds, and an open neural tube defect at the lower spine (arrow). (c) A fragmented embryo (69,XXY) with anencephaly. The arrows indicate an ear and an eye. (d) A fresh embryo (Stage 15) (69,XXX), with no developmental anomalies except for an overgrowth of neural tissue (arrow) above the end of the tail; L, lower limb buds; U, upper limb bud. (e) Typical appearance of cystic villi in triploid early abortuses; cysts, arrows.

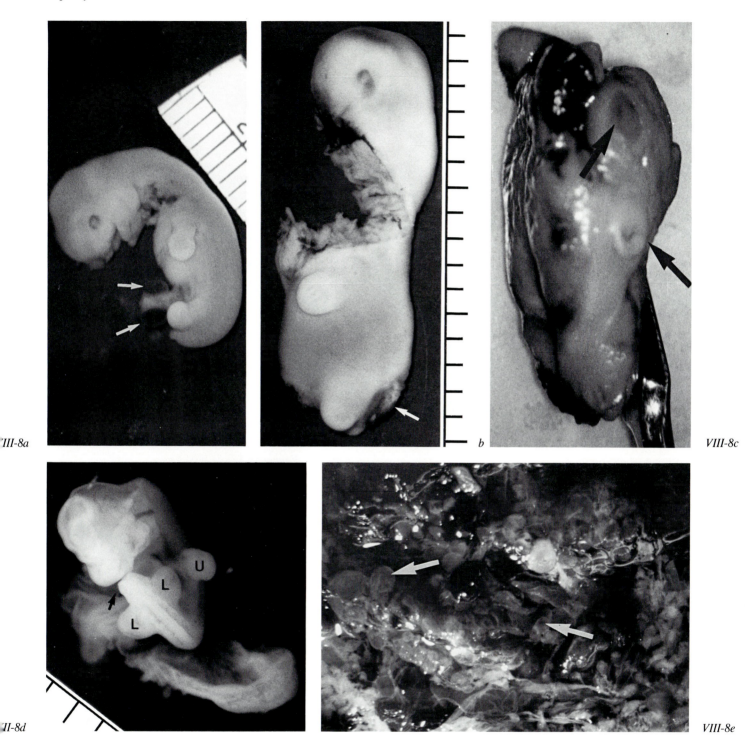

VIII-8a

b

VIII-8c

III-8d

VIII-8e

Tetraploidy

Tetraploidy is less frequent (about 8% of chromosomally abnormal spontaneous abortions) than triploidy and is usually associated with the most severe form of embryonic growth disorganization, intact, empty sacs (Table VIII-2). A frequent finding of amniotic cysts in tetraploid conceptions has been described by Fantel et al. (1980).

Structural Rearrangements

The system for designating structural chromosome aberrations is described in ISCN (1985). Robertsonian and reciprocal translocations are the most frequent rearrangements in humans. Deletions, inversions, and isochromosomes are less common. In early spontaneous abortions, structural rearrangements are relatively uncommon. They can occur de novo as deletions or they can be inherited as unbalanced translocations or derivative chromosomes from a parent who is a carrier of a balanced reciprocal rearrangement. There is an increased frequency of balanced chromosomal rearrangements in infertile couples and couples with recurrent spontaneous abortions. According to different selection criteria, the incidence of chromosomal aberrations in couples with repeated abortions ranges from about 1 to 30% (Pantzar et al., 1984).

The morphology of early abortuses with unbalanced chromosomal rearrangements varies, depending on the degree of genetic imbalance. Embryos with localized defects of face, limbs, or neural tube development represent the most common finding (Table VIII-2), although growth disorganization and completely normal embryonic differentiation are also found. Therefore, morphologic criteria cannot be used to detect spontaneous losses with chromosomal structural defects.

References

Boué J, Boué A, Lazar P: Retrospective and prospective epidemiologic studies of 1500 karyotyped spontaneous human abortions. *Teratology* 12:11–29, 1975.

Fantel AG, Shepard TH, Vadheim-Rok C, Stephens TD, Coleman C: Embryonic and fetal phenotypes. Prevalence and other associated factors in a large study of spontaneous abortion, in Potter IH, Hook EB (eds): *Embryonic and Fetal Death*. New York, Academic Press, 1980, pp 261–287.

Harris M, Poland BJ, Dill FJ: Triploidy in 40 human spontaneous abortuses: Assessment of phenotype in embryos. *Obstet Gynecol* 57:600–609, 1981.

Hertig AT, Rock J, Adams EC: A description of 34 human ova within 17 days of development. *Am J Anat* 98:435–493, 1936.

Honoré LH, Dill FJ, Poland BJ: Placental morphology in spontaneous human abortuses with normal and abnormal karyotypes. *Teratology* 14:151–166, 1976.

ISCN: An international system for human cytogenetic nomenclature. Report of the standing committee on Human Cytogenic Nomenclature. *Cytogenet Cell Genet*, Basel, Karger, 1985.

Jacobs PA, Hassold TJ: Chromosomal abnormalities: Origin and etiology in abortions and live births, in Vogel F, Sperling K (eds): *Human Genetics*. Springer-Verlag, 1987, pp 233–244.

Kalousek DK: Anatomic and chromosomal anomalies in specimens of early spontaneous abortion: Seven year experience. Birth Defects. *OAS* 23:153–168, 1987. New York, Alan R. Liss.

Mall FP: A study of the causes underlying the origin of human monsters. *J Morphol* 19:3–368, 1908.

Pantzar JT, Allanson J, Kalousek D, Poland B: Cytogenetic findings in 318 couples with recurrent spontaneous abortion: A review of experience in British Columbia. *Am J Med Genet* 17:615–620, 1984.

Szulman AE: The biology of trophoblastic disease: Complete and partial hydatidiform mole, in Beard RW, Sharp F (eds): *Early Pregnancy Loss. Mechanisms and Treatment*. Berlin Heidelberg New York, Springer-Verlag, 1988, pp 309–316.

Warburton D, Stein Z, Kline J, Susser M: Chromosome abnormalities in spontaneous abortion, in Porter IH, Hook EB (eds): *Human Embryonic and Fetal Death*. New York, Academic Press, 1980, pp 261–288.

Warburton D, Kline J, Stein Z, Hutzler M, Chin A, Hassolds T: Does the karyotype of a spontaneous abortion predict the karyotype of a subsequent abortion? Evidence from 273 women with two karyotyped spontaneous abortions. *Am J Hum Genet* 41:465–483, 1987.

Fig. VIII-9. Phenotype of tetraploidy: (a) An opened chorionic sac (92,XXYY) with two cystic structures lined by the amnion (C). No embryo, or yolk sac, was identified. (b) An opened chorionic sac with an amnion cyst. No embryo, or yolk sac, identified. (c) A large amnion cyst in an empty chorionic sac.

CHAI

Chr(
Phe)

Introdu

The incide
tions is lo
embryonic
1987). Lat
trisomies g
developme
ploidies ab
may be ret
days to we
the time s
policy to in
ated fetuse
mental def

Most ch
gists are fr
chromoson
appearance
fetus with
prenatal di
niocentesis
20 weeks c
fragmentec
tion is use
following
preserved a
firmatory c
genetic def
phologic fi

Genetic c
mosomal c
somy is nc
aneuploid l
fetuses ter
counseled t

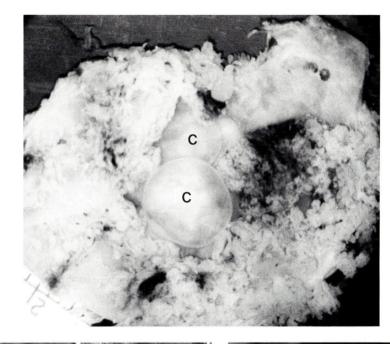

VIII-9a

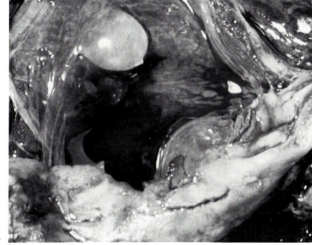

VIII-9b

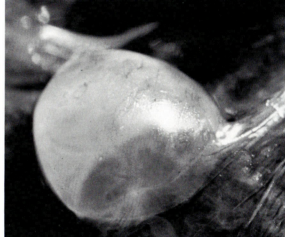

VIII-9c

centesis are usually performed between 16 to 20 weeks of development, and in this group only 22% of the fetuses had nuchal and/or generalized edema. Posterior cervical cystic hygroma may occasionally be present.

Typical craniofacial features seen in newborns with trisomy 21, such as brachycephaly, hypoplasia of the midface, and a flat nasal bridge, are rarely seen in previable fetuses. A flat occiput and upslanting palpebral fissures are seen in about one third to one quarter of the specimens. Brushfield spots of the iris are not developed, and protruding tongue is an uncommon finding. The most frequent external abnormalities in previable fetuses with trisomy 21 are found in the hands and consist of clinodactyly of the fifth fingers, due to hypoplasia or aplasia of the mid-phalanx, and a single palmar crease. Although in normal fetuses (12 to 15 weeks) clinodactyly and a small mid-phalanx of the fifth finger may also be seen, they are usually not present at the time when postamniocentesis therapeutic abortions for trisomy 21 are done. An increased space between the first and second toes is sometimes seen in the fetus before 20 weeks. Femur length is often shortened. This varies from a mild decrease in length to a more marked one; this decrease in femur length is sometimes used as part of the sonographic screening for trisomy 21 (Lockwood et al., 1987; FitzSimmons et al., 1989).

It is not unusual for the fetus with trisomy 21 to have either no external abnormalities (Stephens and Shepard, 1980; Rehder, 1978) or to have only single palmar creases and/or clinodactyly of the fifth fingers. About 10% of trisomy 21 fetuses among our specimens had no external abnormalities, and 29% had only a single palmar crease with or without clinodactyly of the fifth fingers.

Internal development defects are infrequent, except for cardiovascular malformations and abnormal lobation of the lungs. The most common heart abnormalities are atrioven-

tricular canal defects, atrial septal defect (ASD), and ventricular septal defect (VSD). Abnormalities of the vascular system are variable. They include a persistent left superior vena cava, a retroesophageal right subclavian artery, aortic coarctation, and pulmonary stenosis. Although cystic and calcified Hassal corpuscles in the thymus in trisomy 21 appear to be a constant anomaly in older fetuses and newborns (Gilbert et al., 1987), they are not found in previable fetuses.

Multiple anomalies of the brain described in trisomy 21 newborns include brachycephaly, and hypoplasia of the superior temporal gyrus, brainstem, medulla, and cerebellum. None of these defects are usually manifested in the previable trisomy 21 fetuses. Table IX-1 lists the incidence and type of abnormalities present in fetuses with trisomy 21.

TABLE IX.1. Abnormalities in Trisomy 21 Fetuses.

Abnormalities Present in Over 50% of Fetuses	
Clinodactyly of the fifth finger	83%
Absent or small mid-phalanx in the fifth finger after 16 weeks	78%
Heart abnormalities	68%
Abnormalities Present in 10–50% of Fetuses	
Abnormal lobation or fissurization of lungs	47%
Simian crease	38%
Flat occiput	33%
Edema, cystic hygroma, ascites	30%
Abnormal blood vessels (see text)	27%
Upslanting palpebral fissures	22%
Increased space between the first and second toes	20%
Protruding tongue	13%
Lowset ears	10%
Abnormalities present in less than 10% of fetuses see manuscript page 237	

Fig. IX-1. A macerated 9-week fetus (47,XX,+21), showing mild generalized edema.

Fig. IX-2. A spontaneously aborted, 14½-week male fetus (47,XY,+21). Note the posterior cervical hygroma, ascites, and diffuse subcutaneous edema.

Fig. IX-3. (a) A mildly macerated, 17½-week male fetus with sloughing skin (47,XY,+21). Note the simian crease on the right hand. The protruding tongue is an infrequent finding in previable fetuses. (b) Lateral view of the same fetus, showing a flat occiput and a single palmar crease on the right hand.

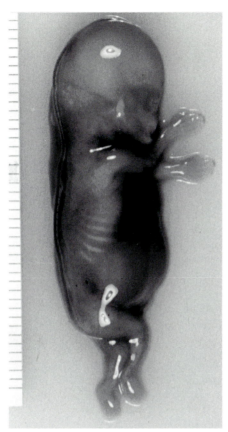

IX-1

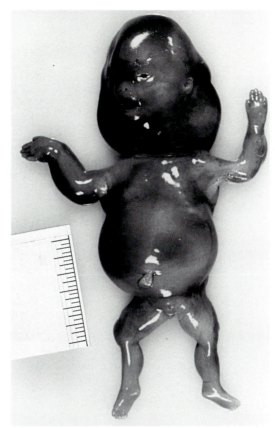

IX-2

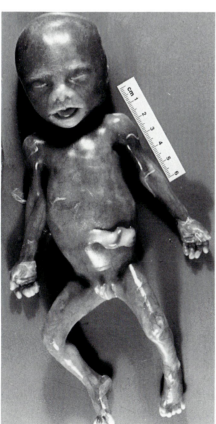

IX-3a

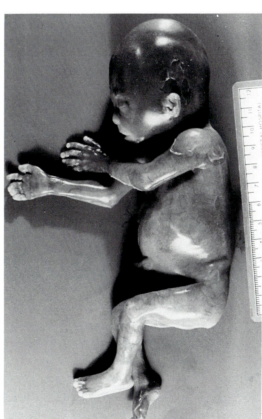

IX-3b

Fig. IX-4. (a) A 19-week male fetus (47,XY,+21) with bilateral simian creases. Note the lack of any "typical" facial features of trisomy 21. (b) A 17½-week female fetus with trisomy 21, showing a complete lack of any typical features of this syndrome.

Fig. IX-5. A 17-week female fetus (47,XY,+21). Note the upslanting palpebral fissures and the increased space between the first and second toes of right foot.

Fig. IX-6. Hand radiogram (magnified) of a 19-week fetus (47,XY,+21) with missing mid-phalangeal bone of the right fifth finger and a tiny mid-phalanx of the left fifth finger.

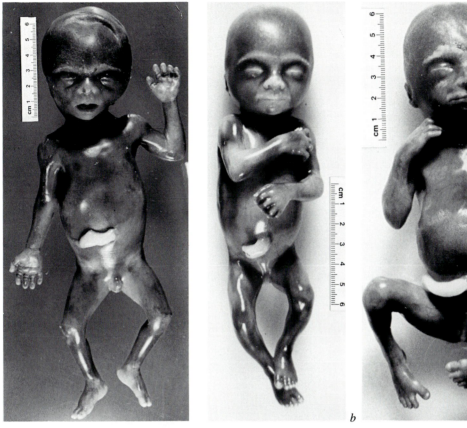

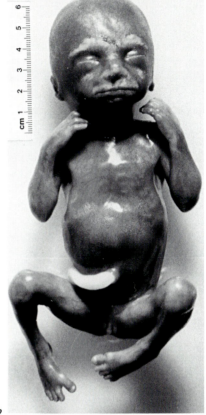

IX-4a

b

IX-5

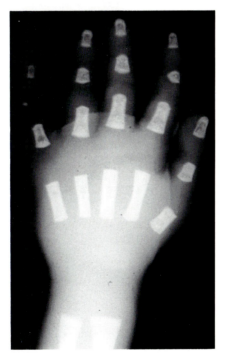

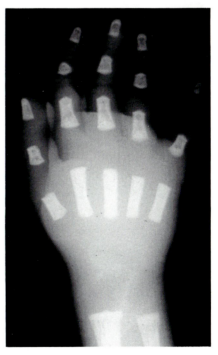

IX-6

Trisomy 18

Trisomy 18 is the second most common chromosomal abnormality found in the newborn population. Fewer than 5% of conceptions with trisomy 18 survive the intrauterine period. About 1.1% of spontaneous abortions and 1.2% of stillbirths have trisomy of chromosome 18 (Jacobs and Hassold, 1987). There are more males in the abortuses and stillbirths and more females in the liveborns. The extra chromosome 18 is present as an additional chromosome in over 80% and as a mosaic in 10%, and it may be found as a translocation in about 5% of trisomic conceptions.

Prenatal growth retardation is the most common finding in trisomy 18 fetuses (Lynch and Berkowitz, 1989). Typical craniofacial features include a triangular face with a small chin. The occiput is not yet prominent and the ears may be low set. In majority of fetuses the appearance of hands and feet is characteristic. The second and fifth fingers usually overlap the third and fourth. This is believed to be due to a displacement of the finger extensor tendons over the metacarpophalangeal joints (Pettersen and Bersu, 1982) and is not seen in macerated fetuses or before 14 weeks of gestation. In the lateral view, the feet have prominent heels and a rocker-bottom appearance, due to vertical taluses in one third of fetuses. Cardiac defects are nearly always present, with polyvalvular dysplasia being the most frequent finding (van Praagh et al., 1989). Omphalocele and renal abnormalities are common. Neural tube defects may be found but are not common (Matsuoka et al., 1981).

No difference in the type or frequency of abnormalities found in the spontaneously and the therapeutically aborted group has been found (McFadden and Kalousek, personal communication).

Table IX-2 lists the incidence and type of abnormalities present in fetuses with trisomy 18.

Fig. IX-7. A macerated, spontaneously aborted, 10½-week male fetus (47,XY, +18) with mild neck edema and an omphalocele.

Fig. IX-8. A macerated, 12½-week male fetus (47,XY, +18) with no external developmental defects—ventricular septal defect and pulmonary hypoplasia were found on internal examination.

Fig. IX-9. A lateral view of a macerated, 14½-week male fetus (47,XY, +18) with a cystic hygroma, a cleft lip on the right side, and marked generalized edema. Overlapping fingers are not usually seen in macerated fetuses.

Fig. IX-10. A 17-week female fetus (47,XY, +18). Note the globular head, small face, micrognathia, overlapping fingers, and a small umbilical hernia containing two loops of small bowel.

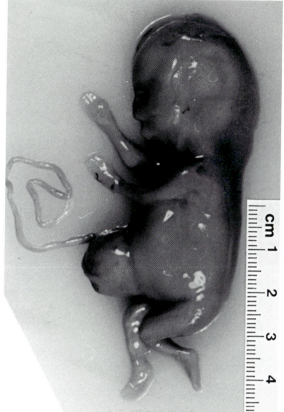

IX-7

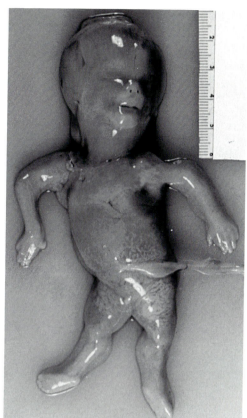

IX-8

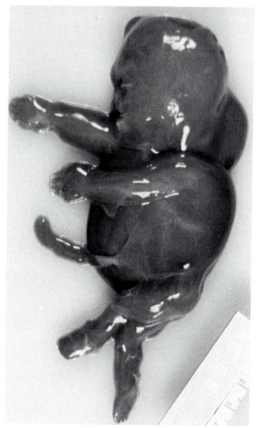

IX-9

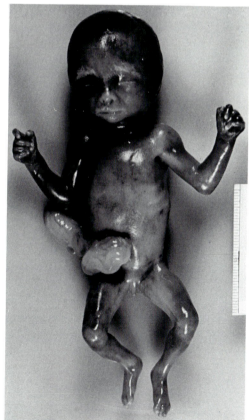

IX-10

TABLE IX.2. Abnormalities in Trisomy 18 Fetuses.

Head and Face
Micrognathia	29%
Low-set ears	25%
Triangular face	21%
Cleft lip and/or palate	12%
Small mouth	8%
Prominent occiput	4%
Preauricular tag	4%
Absent external ear	4%
Epicanthus	4%

Neck
Cystic hygroma, edema	25%

Extremities
Fingers two and five overlap fingers three and four	50%
Rocker bottom feet	33%
Clinodactyly of the fifth finger	21%
Clubfeet	17%
Joint contractures, with webbing	12%
Duplicated or absent thumb	12%
Short arms	8%

Cardiovascular System
Any heart defect	96%
Polyvalvular dysplasia	62%
Aortic coarctation	21%
Ventricular septal defect	19%
Atrial septal defect	17%
Persistent left superior vena cava	17%
Retroesophageal subclavian artery	12%
Hypoplastic left ventricle	4%
Atrioventricular canal	4%

Respiratory System
Abnormal lobation of lungs	37%
Hypoplasia of lungs	12%

Gastrointestinal System
Omphalocele	33%
Meckel's diverticulum	12%
Gut malrotation	12%
Tracheoesophageal fistula	12%

Urogenital System
Horseshoe kidney	33%
Kidney hypoplasia	8%
Dilated ureter	8%
Double ureter	8%
Bifurcated ureter	4%
Enlarged kidney	4%
Small penis	4%
Bicornuate uterus	4%

Meningomyelocele	4%
Spleen Hypoplasia	4%
Adrenal Hypoplasia	4%
Thymus Hypoplasia	4%
Eventration of diaphragm	20%

Fig. IX-11. A 19-week female fetus (48,XXX,+18) with overlapping fingers, micrognathia, and extended legs.

Fig. IX-12. A 16-week male fetus (47,XY,+18) with bilateral club hands. Both the radius and ulna are present. Note the rounded head, micrognathia, and prominent heels.

Fig. IX-13. A close up of the hands, showing the typical positioning of the second over the third and the fifth over the fourth finger on the left hand. The right hand shows only an overlapping of the second and third finger. The hands are from 18-week female fetus (47,XX,+18).

Fig. IX-14. Dysplastic tricuspid valve (D), with blood cysts (B), from a 17-week fetus (47,XX,+18); V, right ventricle; A, right atrium.

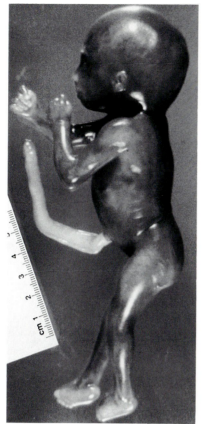

IX-11

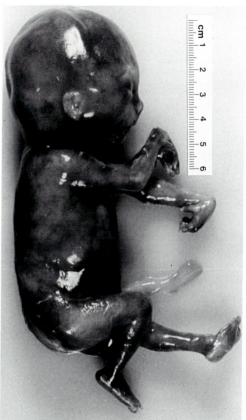

IX-12

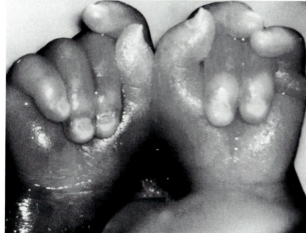

IX-13

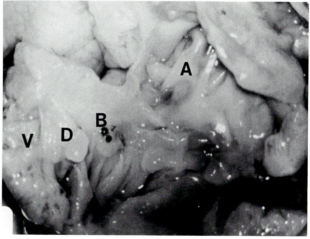

IX-14

Trisomy 13

Trisomy 13 is present in about 0.005 of liveborns and in 1.1% of spontaneously aborted conceptuses; 97% of conceptions with trisomy 13 die before birth (Jacobs and Hassold, 1987). The extra chromosome 13 can be present as an additional chromosome or, in 20% of cases, as a translocation.

Most of the abnormalities typical of trisomy 13 newborns are present in the previable fetus as well (Jones, 1988). Craniofacial abnormalities include holoprosencephalic-type defects, microcephaly, microphthalmia, cleft lip and/or palate, and scalp defects. Postaxial polydactyly in one or more limbs and cardiac abnormalities are usually present. Neural tube defects, malrotation of the intestine, with or without omphalocele, and such variable renal anomalies as microcysts involving nephrons and collecting tubules, nodular renal blastema, and renal dysplasia are commonly seen. Fujinaga et al. (1989) reported increased kidney weights in eight of nine fetuses, and ectopic or accessory spleens are often seen (Hashida et al., 1983). Compared to other autosomal trisomies, fetuses with trisomy 13 show more severe craniofacial, skeletal, and brain abnormalities. No difference in the type or incidence of abnormalities has been observed in trisomy 13 fetuses spontaneously or therapeutically aborted (McFadden and Kalousek, personal communication).

There are detailed histopathologic descriptions of lesions of the eye, such as retinal dysplasia, uveal tract colobomas, and intraocular cartilage, in older fetuses (Gilbert et al., 1987), as well as dysplastic cerebellar heterotopias and pancreatic dysplasia (Moerman et al., 1988). These have not been observed in previable fetuses.

Table IX-3 reports the incidence and type of abnormalities found in fetuses with trisomy 13.

TABLE IX.3. Abnormalities in Trisomy 13 Fetuses.

Head and Face	
Microcephaly	55%
Hypoplastic or absent nose	55%
Cleft lip and palate	55%
Small eyes	44%
Low-set ears	33%
Hypotelorism	33%
Holoprosencephaly	22%
Parietal scalp defect	11%
Abnormally shaped ears	11%
Cyclopia	11%
Encephalocoele	11%
Absent uvula	11%
Neck	
Edema	11%
Extremities	
Postaxial polydactyly (hands)	77%
Postaxial polydactyly (feet)	11%
Cardiovascular System	
Any heart defect	77%
Tetralogy of Fallot	33%
Ventricular septal defect and atrial septal defect	22%
Isolated VSD	22%
Double outlet right ventricle	11%
Mitral valve atresia	11%
Bicuspid aortic valve	11%
Respiratory System	
Abnormal lobation of lungs	55%
Hypoplasia of lungs	33%
Abnormal fissurization of lungs	22%
Gastrointestinal System	
Malrotation of the small bowel	33%
Meckel's diverticulum	11%
Umbilical hernia or omphalocele	11%
Urogenital System	
Small penis	50%
Horseshoe kidney	22%
Enlarged kidneys (unexplained)	11%
Hydronephrosis	11%
Extra Splenic Tissue	22%
Meningomyelocele or myelocele	20%

Fig. IX-15. The head of a macerated, fragmented 9-week male fetus (47,XY, +13). The craniofacial anomalies include microcephaly, a proboscis (arrow), and cyclopia (C).

Fig. IX-16. A macerated, 9-week female fetus (47,XX, +13). Note the microphthalmia, hypotelorism, hypoplastic nose, and left unilateral cleft lip.

Fig. IX-17. A posterior view of a degenerated, 9-week female fetus (47,XX, +13), showing bilateral polydactyly (arrows) and a lumbosacral myelocele.

Fig. IX-18. A 16½-week male fetus (47,XY, +13) with bilateral postaxial polydactyly of the hands and a small penis. Note the lack of characteristic facial features.

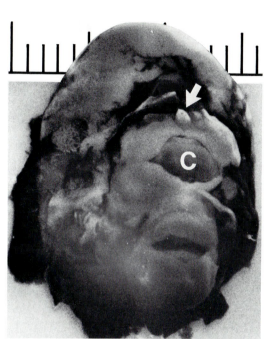

IX-15

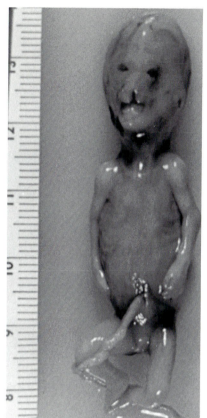

IX-16

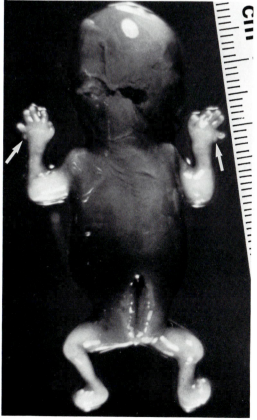

IX-17

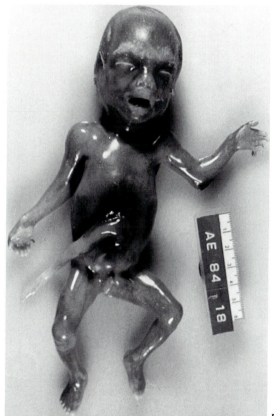

IX-18

Fig. IX-19. A 17-week male fetus (47,XY,+13) with cebocephaly, holoprosencephaly, and a small penis. Internal examination revealed cardiac defects and pulmonary hypoplasia.

Fig. IX-20. (a) A 18-week male fetus (47,XY,+13). Note the microcephaly, hypotelorism, absent nose, and a large median cleft lip. A cleft palate is also present. (b) The same fetus as shown in Figure IX-20a. Note the microcephaly and postaxial polydactyly of both hands. (c) The same fetus as shown in Figure IX-20a. Note the scalp defect (arrow) and postaxial polydactyly of both hands.

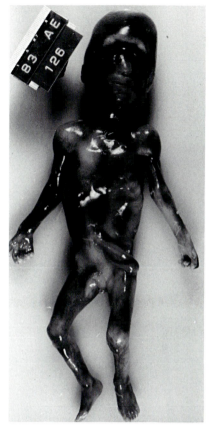

IX-19

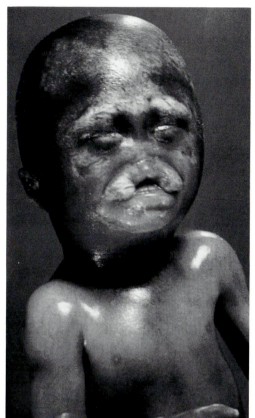

IX-20a

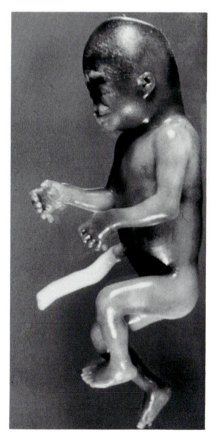

IX-20b

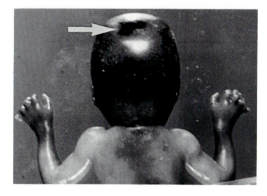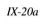

IX-20c

Monosomy X

Monosomy X is the most common chromosome defect among second trimester abortuses. About 10% of all abortuses are 45,X, and fewer than 5% of conceptions with monosomy X survive until birth (Jacobs and Hassold, 1987).

The appearance of the spontaneously aborted 45,X fetus before 20 weeks is very different from the 45,X newborn. Such 45,X fetuses usually have a large posterior nuchal cystic hygroma, with generalized edema and hypoplasia of the preductal aortic arch. It is been postulated that generalized edema and cystic hygroma are the result of hypoplasia and/or aplasia of the lymphatic vessels and a failure of the jugular lymph sacs and the jugular vein to communicate (Van der Putte, 1977). Most abnormalities typical of the newborn—a broad chest with widely spaced nipples, anomalous auricles, a low posterior hairline, a short webbed neck, narrow fingernails, and dorsal lymphedema in the hands and feet—appear to represent sequelae of fetal edema and cystic hygroma. It has been suggested (Clark, 1984; Lacroe et al., 1988) that preductal aortic hypoplasia may also be secondary to altered blood flow caused by lymphatic underdevelopment.

Posterior cervical hygroma has been described in many genetic and nongenetic syndromes. These include trisomies 13, 18, and 21; lethal multiple pterygium syndrome; Noonan syndrome; Roberts syndrome; and Cowchock syndrome. However, in 45,X fetuses, cervical hygroma is always accompanied by generalized edema and preductal aortic hypoplasia, which is not true for other conditions with cystic hygroma (Kalousek and Seller, 1987). Another important difference in lymphatic vessel development between fetuses with 45,X and fetuses with some other conditions seems to be that, in the 45,X fetuses, the lymph vessels throughout the body are both dilated and decreased in number, whereas in some other conditions, the lymph vessels are dilated but increased in number (Chitayat et al., 1988).

Although the main feature of adults with 45,X is infertility,

TABLE IX.4. Abnormalities in 45,X Fetuses.

Abnormalities Present in Over 50% of Fetuses	
Nuchal cystic hygroma or nuchal edema	100%
Generalized edema	100%
Hypoplasia of preductal aortic arch	100%
Incomplete lung lobation or fissurization	62%
Horseshoe kidney	52%
Abnormalities Present in 10–50% of Fetuses	
Bicuspid aortic valve	38%
Persistent left superior vena cava	19%
Malrotation of the bowel	19%
Ascites	14%
Abnormalities Present in Less Than 10% of Fetuses	
Hypoplasia of the left common iliac artery, ventricular septal defect, left ventricle hypoplasia, mitral valve stenosis, tricuspid valve hyperplasia, abnormal pulmonary valve, single coronary ostium, Meckel's diverticulum, short small bowel, hemidiaphragm, hypoplastic kidney, hydroureter, ectopic kidney, and omphalocele	

due to streak gonads, some ova were identified in all the ovaries from 10- to 20-week fetuses. It is difficult to evaluate accurately the decrease in number of ova in ovaries of aborted fetuses, since the tissue is frequently autolyzed and/or otherwise damaged. It has been postulated that ova in 45,X fetuses develop normally but that impaired follicular development due to the absence of the second X chromosome leads to gradual loss of ova during gestation and the development of the small fibrotic ovaries that are seen in 45,X newborns.

Table IX-4 lists abnormalities found in 45,X fetuses. Although many different chromosome abnormalities, such as X chromosome deletions or X chromosome rearrangements, can produce the adult Turner syndrome phenotype characterized by infertility with or without short stature, it is not clear whether and to what degree these abnormalities affect fetal phenotype.

Fig. IX-21. A macerated, 11-week 45,X fetus with a large posterior cervical nuchal cystic hygroma and generalized edema.

Fig. IX-22. A 15-week 45,X fetus. Note the nuchal cystic hygroma and generalized edema, which is especially pronounced on the dorsum of the hands and feet (arrows).

Fig. IX-23. A macerated, 15-week 45,X fetus with generalized edema and a large nuchal cystic hygroma expanding anteriorly.

Fig. IX-24. Collected parts of a fragmented 14.5-week fetus, with four identified extremities, a collapsed skull, and no internal organs, terminated after an ultrasound diagnosis of amniotic band syndrome. Note the marked dorsal edema of both feet (arrows) and the upper arm, suggestive of monosomy X. No cytogenetic diagnosis is available because the culture was infected.

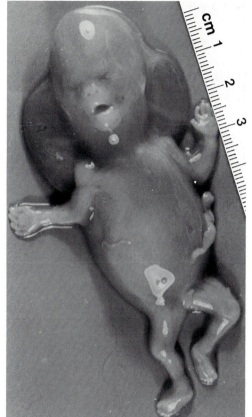

IX-21

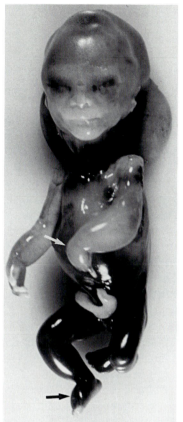

IX-22

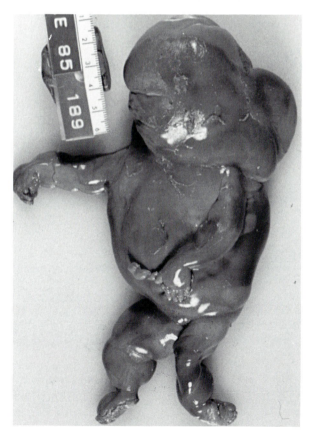

IX-23

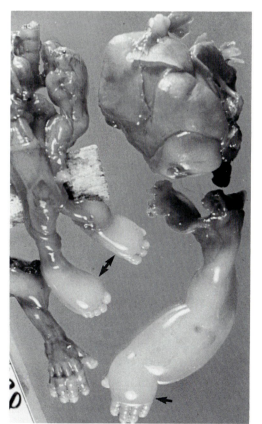

IX-24

Triploidy

Appoximately 7.3% of all spontaneous aborted fetuses and 0.6% of stillborns have an extra set of chromosomes, that is, they are triploid. Very few triploid conceptuses survive until birth (Jacobs and Hassold, 1987).

Triploidy may result from a number of different mechanisms, including dispermy, fusion of a diploid sperm with a haploid oocyte, or fertilization of a diploid oocyte by a haploid sperm. The most common event is dispermy (Niebuhr, 1974).

The extra set of chromosomes can be either of paternal or maternal origin. If the supernumerary set is paternal, placental changes characteristic of partial hydatidiform moles are usually found; if the extra set is maternal, the placenta is usually small and fibrotic (Jacobs et al., 1982). The majority of triploid abortions in the previable fetal period show a placental phenotype that is consistent with a maternal origin of the extra set. This contrasts with the embryonic triploidy loss, which shows mainly placental phenotype consistent with a paternal origin of the extra set.

Most triploid fetuses show severe intrauterine growth retardation. They have large heads, a cleft palate, syndactyly between the third and the fourth fingers, and heart defects. Ambiguous genitalia are common among those with a 69,XXY karyotype. The typical phenotype of fetal triploidy, with severe intrauterine growth retardation and a large fetal head, includes a small fibrotic placenta. Preliminary findings indicate that these fetuses arise from a double maternal complement and a single paternal one (McFadden and Kalousek, 1990). It is interesting to note that the more rare, large cystic placentas are usually seen with the microcephalic, well-nourished triploid fetus. These fetuses originate from a double paternal and a single maternal complement. There seems to be no difference in type and frequency of internal developmental defects between maternally and paternally derived triploid fetuses.

The observed abnormalities and their incidence in the triploid fetuses are listed in Table IX-5.

TABLE IX.5. Abnormalities in Triploid Fetuses.

Head and Face	
Large head	75%
Cleft palate	50%
Low-set ears	25%
Small mandible	25%
Cleft lip	16%
Small head	16%
Single ventricle in brain	8%
Microphthalmia or opaque lens	8%
Large ears	8%
Jaw synechiae	8%
Neck	
Edema	16%
Extremities	
Syndactyly between the third and the fourth fingers	58%
Clinodactyly of the fifth finger	16%
Contractures of the wrists and fingers	8%
Hypoplastic thumb	8%
Syndactyly between the toes	50%
Cardiovascular System	
Any heart defect	66%
Atrial septal defect and ventricular septal defect	25%
Ventricular septal defect isolated	25%
Valve dysplasia	25%
Atrioventricular canal	16%
Aortic stenosis	16%
Single ventricle	8%
Double outlet right ventricle	8%
Respiratory System	
Hypoplastic lungs	66%
Abnormal lobation/fissurization of lungs	66%
Gastrointestinal System	
Malrotation of small bowel	33%
Short large bowel	8%
Imperforate anus	8%
Liver hypoplasia	8%
Urogenital System	
Ambiguous genitalia	58%
Hypoplastic kidney	8%
Horseshoe kidney	8%
Adrenal Gland	
Severe hypoplasia	75%
Lumbrosacral Neural Tube Defect	16%
Hirsutism	8%
Placenta	
Cystic dilation of placental villi	8%
Small placenta	92%
Oligohydramnios	16%

Fig. IX-25. (a) A macerated, 12½-week fetus (69,XXX). Note the large head, low-set ears, finger syndactyly, and general reduction in muscle volume. The neck appears enlarged due to the angle of the photograph. (b) A lateral view of the same fetus showing, in addition, an open neural tube defect in the lumbosacral region (arrow).

Fig. IX-26. A macerated, 12½-week fetus, with 69,XXY complement. Note the syndactyly of fingers three and four (arrow), poorly developed muscle tissue, and the small placenta. Focal swelling of the umbilical cord is due to autolysis.

Fig. IX-27. A lateral view of a well-preserved, 15-week fetus (69,XXY). Note the large head, small mandible, small face, and poorly developed muscle. Arrow points to syndactyly of fingers three and four.

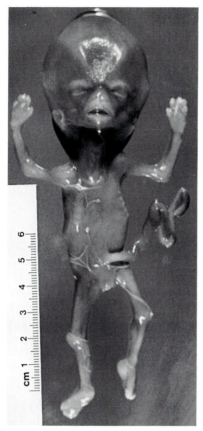
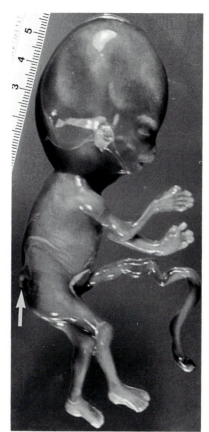
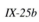

IX-25a   *IX-25b*

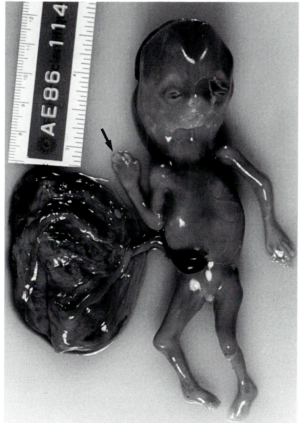
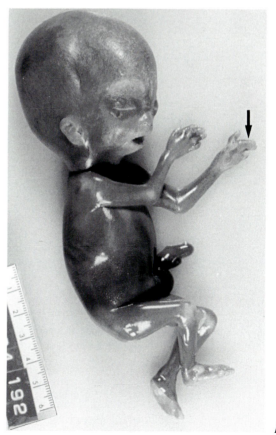

IX-26   *IX-27*

Fig. IX-28. A macerated, 8-week female fetus (69,XXX). Note the absence of any external developmental defects. Internal anomalies included an atrioventricular canal, a horseshoe kidney, hypoplastic adrenals and lungs, and bowel malrotation.

Fig. IX-29. The adrenals and kidneys from a 13-week fetus (69,XXX). Note the severe adrenal hypoplasia.

Fig. IX-30. (a) A 15-week fetus (69,XXX) and a large placenta. Note the different fetal phenotype with microcephaly and relatively well-developed muscle tissue. (b) The maternal placental surface, showing multiple cysts; arrows, large cysts.

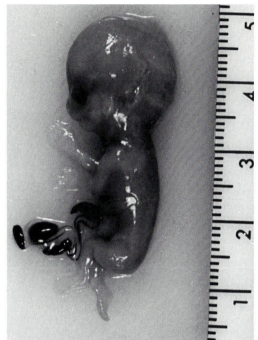
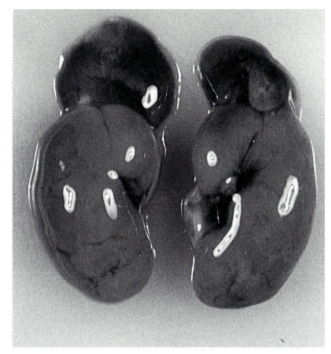

IX-28

IX-29

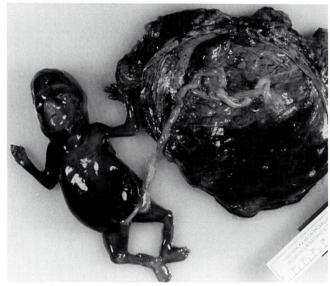
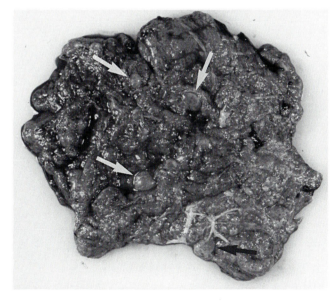

IX-30a

IX-30b

47,XXX

About 0.1% of spontaneous abortuses, 0.3% of stillbirths, and 0.05% of live births are females with an additional X chromosome. The majority of XXX females have no recognizable physical abnormalities, and most newborns are normal except for clinodactyly and epicanthic folds which are increased in frequency in these newborn (Robinson et al., 1979).

Our experience confirms that normal development is also observed among fetuses terminated for prenatal diagnosis of 47,XXX. The histology of the ovaries usually was normal in

TABLE IX.6. Abnormalities in 47,XXX Fetuses.

Bilateral clinodactyly of the fifth finger	20%
Abnormal lung lobation	10%
Flat occiput	10%
Low-set ears	10%
Small narrow ureter, dysplastic multicystic kidney	10%

our group of XXX females and has been so reported (Autio-Harmainen et al., 1980).

Table IX-6 lists the low incidence and limited types of abnormalities found in 47,XXX examined fetuses.

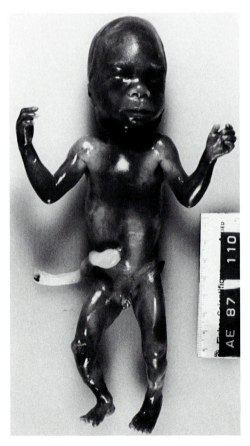 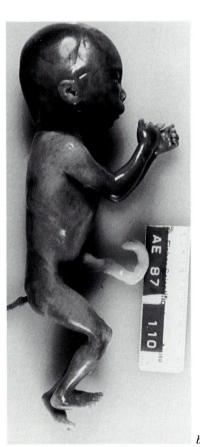 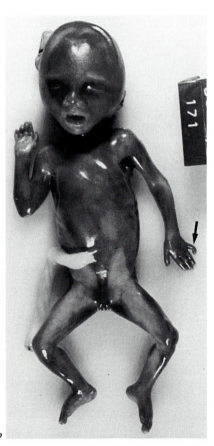

IX-31a   b   IX-32

Fig. IX-31. (a) A 17-week fetus (47,XXX). Note the normal appearance. (b) Lateral view of the same fetus. Note the prolapse of the large bowel secondary to pregnancy termination.

Fig. IX-32. A 17-week fetus (47,XXX). No developmental defects, except for a bilateral clinodactyly of the fifth finger (arrow), are seen.

47,XXY

Klinefelter syndrome (47,XXY) is the most common cause of male hypogonadism and infertility. It is present in 0.2% of all spontaneous aborted fetuses and 0.4% of stillborns; 96% of conceptuses with 47,XXY survive until birth.

As most XXY fetuses are normal, uterine or placental pathology is the major cause of spontaneous abortions in this group.

A major congenital abnormality was found in 18% of XXY newborns. The most frequent abnormalities were cleft palate, inguinal hernia, and testis retention. Minor abnormalities were found in 26% of these newborns; the most frequent was clinodactyly, but there is no clear-cut pattern of abnormalities (Robinson et al., 1979).

Testicular morphology has been reported in three fetuses, 16 to 20 weeks of gestation. In two cases the testes were normal, but the third had hyperplasia of the Leydig cells, hypoplastic tubules, and severely reduced germinal epithelium (Murken et al., 1974; Rock et al., 1982).

TABLE IX.7. Abnormalities in 47,XXY Fetuses.

Hypospadias involving only the glans	10%
Testicular abnormality:	10%
slight increase in the number of Leydig cells	
reduction in the number of germ cells or reduction in	
the size of the seminiferous tubules	
Clinodactyly of the fifth finger	10%
Meckel's diverticulum	10%

Table IX-7 reports the incidence and types of abnormalities found in these fetuses.

47,XYY

About 0.11% of newborn males are XYY. These newborns are normal in appearance. However, there have been two reports of abnormal brain development. Brun and Gustavson (1972) described a boy with a megalencephalic brain and mild cortical dysplasia, diffuse neuronal heterotopias of white matter, and signs of retarded cellular maturation. A 21-week-old fetus was

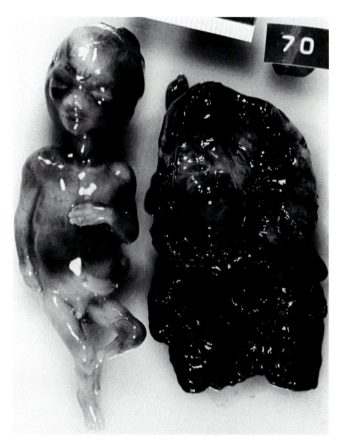
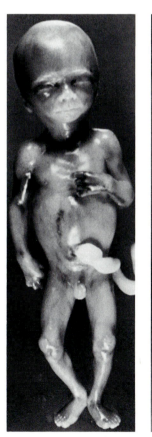
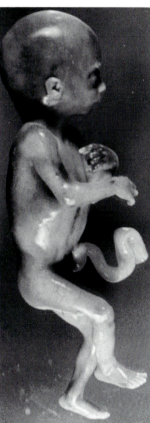

IX33   a   IX-34b

Fig. IX-33. A 12½-week fetus (47,XXY) spontaneously aborted due to intrauterine infection and retroplacental hemorrhage. Note the normal appearance of the fetus.

Fig. IX-34. (a) A 19-week fetus (47,XXY). Note the normal appearance. (b) Lateral view of the same fetus.

found to have an abnormal pattern of cerebral convolutions (Austin and Sparkes, 1980). These observations may be no more than coincidental, and further documentation of this association is needed. Fetal gonadal histology is normal.

Structural Chromosome Rearrangements

Structural rearrangements can be balanced or unbalanced. Whereas balanced translocations are compatible with normal intrauterine development, unbalanced translocations (partial duplications or partial deletions) may produce developmental defects and intrauterine death (Schinzel, 1984). Intrauterine death, however, is rarely seen in the previable fetal period and is more common in the perinatal period. Both balanced and unbalanced chromosomal rearrangements can be detected by cytogenetic prenatal diagnosis. Morphologic findings in fetuses with unbalanced chromosomal rearrangement vary, depending on the amount and type of genetic material lost or duplicated. Abnormal morphologic findings are usually absent when the rearrangement appears to be balanced. It is the reported increased risk of mental retardation in the individuals with balanced translocations that makes some families decide for pregnancy termination in cases of prenatal detection of a balanced translocation (Fryns et al., 1986).

References

Austin G, Sparkes R: Abnormal cerebral cortical convolutions in an XYY fetus. *Hum Genet* 56:173–175, 1980.

Autio-Harmainen H, Rapola J, Aula P: Fetal gonadal histology in XXXXY, XYY and XXX syndromes. *Clin Gen* 18:1–5, 1980.

Brun A, Gustavson K: Cerebral malformations in the XYY syndrome. *Acta Pathol Microbiol Scand* (Section A) 80:627–633, 1972.

Chitayat D, Kalousek D, Bamforth J: The lymphatic abnormalities in fetuses with posterior cervical cystic hygroma. *Am J Med Genet* 33:352–356, 1989.

Clark E: Neck web and congenital heart defects: A pathogenic association in 45 X-O Turner's syndrome? *Teratology* 29:355–361, 1984.

Craver RD, Kalousek DK: Cytogenetic abnormalities among spontaneously aborted previable fetuses. *Am J Med Genet* (Suppl 3):113–119, 1987.

FitzSimmons J, Droste S, Shepard TH, Pascoe-Mason J, Chinn A, Mack LA: Long-bone growth in fetuses with Down syndrome. *Am J Obstet Gynecol* 161:1174–1177.

Fryns J, Kleczowska A, Kubien E, Van den Berghe H: Excess of mental retardations and/or congenital malformation in reciprocal translocations in man. *Hum Genet* 72:1–8, 1986.

Fujinaga M, Shepard T, Fitzsimmons J: Trisomy 13 in the fetus. *Teratology* 39:454, 1989.

Gilbert EF, Arya S, Laxova R, Opitz J: Pathology of chromosome abnormalities in the fetus—pathologic markers. *Birth Defects OAS* 23:293–306, 1987.

Hashida Y, Jaffe R, Huni EJ: Pancreatic pathology in trisomy 13: Specificity of the morphologic lesion. *Pediatr Pathol* 1:169–178, 1983.

Jacobs PA, Hassold TJ: Chromosome abnormalities: Origin and etiology in abortions and live births, in Vogel F, Sperling K (eds): *Human Genetics*. Berlin, Springer-Verlag, 1987, pp 233–244.

Jacobs P, Szulman A, Funkhouser J, Matsuura J, Wilson C: Human triploidy: Relationship between paternal origin of the additional haploid complement and development of partial hydatidiform mole. *Ann Hum Genet* 46:223–231, 1982.

Jones K: *Smith's Recognizable Patterns of Human Malformation*, ed 4. Philadelphia, WB Saunders, 1988.

Kalousek D, Seller M: Differential diagnosis of posterior cervical hygroma in previable fetuses. *Am J Med Genet* (suppl) 3:83–92, 1987.

Lacro R, Jones K, Benirschke K: Coarctation of the aorta in Turner syndrome. *Pediatrics* 81:445–451, 1988.

Lockwood C, Benacerraf B, Kinsky A, Blakemore K, Belanger K, Mahoney M, Hobbins J: A sonographic screening method for Down syndrome. *Am J Obstet Gynol* 157:803–808, 1987.

Lynch L, Berkowitz RL: First trimester growth delay in trisomy 18. *Am J Perinatol* 6:237–239, 1989.

McFadden D, Kalousek D: Fetal triploid phenotypes: Correlation with parental origin of extra haploid set. *Am J Med Genet* in press.

Matsuoka R, Matsuyama S, Yamamoto Y, Kuroki Y, Matsui I: Trisomy 18q. A case report and review of karyotype-phenotype correlations. *Hum Genet* 57:78–82, 1981.

Moerman P, Fryns J-P, van der Steen K, Kleczkowska A, Lauweryns J: The pathology of trisomy 13 syndrome. A study of 12 cases. *Hum Genet* 80:349–356, 1988.

Murken J, Stengel-Rutkowski S, Walthier J, Westenfelder S, Remberger K, Zimmer R: Klinefelter's syndrome in a fetus. *Lancet* i:171, 1984.

Niebuhr E: Triploidy in man. *Humangenetik* 21:103–125, 1974.

Pettersen JC, Bersu ET: A comparison of the anatomical variations found in trisomes 13, 18 and 21, in Persaud E (ed): *Genetic Disorders, Syndromology and Prenatal Diagnosis*. Lancaster, MTP Press, 1982, pp 161–179.

Rehder M: Embryopathology in prenatal diagnosis, in Murker JD (ed): *Prenatal Diagnosis*. Stuttgart, Ferdinand Enke, 1978, pp 336–341.

Robinson A, Lubs H, Nielsen J, Sorensen K: Summary of clinical findings: Profiles of children with 47,XXY, 47,XXX and 47,XYY karyotypes. *Birth Defects* OAS XV 1:261–266, 1979.

Rock J, Rock W, Rary J: Testicular morphology in the 47,XXY fetus at 16 weeks gestation. *Int J Gynaecol Obstetr* 20:261–263, 1982.

Schinzel A: *Catalogue of Unbalanced Chromosome Aberrations in Man*. Berlin, de Gruyter, 1984.

Stephens T, Shepard T: The Down syndrome in the fetus. *Teratology* 22:37–41, 1980.

Van der Putte S: Lymphatic malformation in human fetuses. A study of fetuses with Turner's syndrome or status Bonnevie-Ullrich. *Virchows Arch* (Pathol Anat) 376:233–246, 1977.

Van Praagh S, Truman T, Firpo A, Bano-Rodrigo A, Fried R, McManus B, Engle MA, Van Praagh R: Cardiac malformations in trisomy-18: A study of 41 postmortem cases. *J Am Coll Cardiol* 13:1586–1597, 1989.

Warburton D, Kline J, Stein Z, Hutzler M, Chin A, Hassold T: Does the karyotype of a spontaneous abortion predict the karyotype of a subsequent abortion? *Am J Hum Genet* 41:465–487, 1987.

CHAPTER X

Placental Abnormalities

Introduction

All placentas from spontaneous abortions should be submitted for pathologic examination. The placenta plays a key role in the maintenance of pregnancy, and it is likely that it also is a major influence on the processes involved in expulsion of an aborting conceptus. For example, it has been shown that fetuses with trisomy 13 and 18 that survive to term have confined chromosomal mosaicism, with a normal diploid cell line in the cytotrophoblast (Kalousek et al., 1989). Chromosomally normal fetuses with confined placental mosaicism involving various trisomies are more likely to die in utero (Johnson et al., 1990). Because of the key role of the placenta at its interface with the maternal organism, it follows that detailed studies may provide valuable data on both intrauterine fetal survival and mechanisms of spontaneous abortion.

Many authors address the topic of proper placental examination (Boyd and Hamilton, 1970; Fox, 1978; Altshuler, 1981; Perrin and Sander, 1984). Briefly, placentas should be examined while they are still fresh, to allow sampling for microbiologic, cytogenetic, electron microscopic, and metabolic studies when necessary. Each placental component (membranes, cord, and placental disc) should be examined for the presence of developmental defects and pathologic lesions. After its appearance has been described, the cord and membranes are removed and the placenta is weighed; the disc should be sliced at 1-cm intervals or less. Histologic sections should be taken from the cord, membranes, and the placental disc, the number dictated by the types and number of abnormalities observed. Both normal-appearing parenchyma and any lesion should be examined histologically.

The most common findings in the placentas of previable fetuses are summarized below. For the pathology of the early chorionic sac, see Chapter IV.

Extraembryonic Membranes

Amnion Cysts

Amnion cysts observed early in gestation are usually associated with chromosomal tetraploidy (see Chapter VIII). They vary in size from a few millimeters to 2 to 3 cm. They are filled with a clear amniotic fluid and lined by amnion. Their attachment to the rest of the amnion is usually broad. In anembryonic sacs, the cysts orientation is difficult to establish. When an embryo is present, they are usually found near the insertion of the cord.

Amnion-Chorion Fusion

Amnion-chorion fusion normally occurs from 10 to 12 weeks of gestation but occurs earlier when embryonic growth disorganization is present (see Chapter IV and VI). The persistence of an extraembryonic celom and a lack of amnion-chorion fusion has been described by van Allen et al. (1987) for fetuses with the limb body wall complex.

Amnion Rupture

Amnion rupture sequence with amniotic bands and the limb body wall complex are described as the most common consequences of amnion rupture prior to 20 weeks of gestation (Chapter VI).

Amnion Nodosum

Amnion nodosum, a nodular outcrop on the amnion surface, consists of deposits of vernix caseosa and degenerated epithelial cells of fetal and amniotic origin, which are attached to areas of denudation of amniotic epithelium. A complication of severe oligohydramnios, it is due to impaired fetal urine production. Amnion nodosum is a rare finding in previable gestations because the concentration of cellular elements in amniotic fluid prior to 20-weeks of gestation is low.

Chorioamnionitis

The placenta of about one third of spontaneously aborted fresh fetuses shows chorioamnionitis. This represents a response of the maternal and/or fetal polymorphonuclear leukocytes to chemotactic substances from infectious organisms that have ascended to enter the amniotic cavity. It is not always clear whether this lesion is causal or coincidental with the abortion (e.g., in cervical insufficiency). For a detailed description and illustrations, see Chapter VII.

Umbilical Cord

Abnormal Length of the Cord

There are no adequate data on the normal length variation of the umbilical cord during the embryonic and previable period. Cord measurements collected from 93 normal previable fetuses are shown in Appendix II, Table II-5. At the end of the previable period, the average length of the cord is from 21 to 23 cm.

The cord may appear thin, long, and excessively spiraled in retained macerated conceptuses.

A short cord is a well-established pathologic entity (Grange et al., 1987). It is always found in gestations in which the mobility of the embryo or fetus is significantly reduced, such as in the limb body wall complex (Chapter VI) or the multiple pterygium syndrome (Chapter VI). It may also be associated with omphalocele and has been observed in cases of severe oligohydramnios.

Vestigial Remnants

Remnants of the allantoic or omphalomesenteric ducts may be apparent on microscopic examination of the cord, particularly in sections taken near the fetal end. Allantoic remnants are usually seen between the two umbilical arteries and appear either as a solid cord or as a duct lined by flattened or transitional epithelium. Remnants of the omphalomesenteric duct are usually situated at the margin of the cord and are lined by cuboidal or columnar epithelium (see Chapter VI).

Single Umbilical Artery

The incidence of a single umbilical artery in perinatal autopsy studies has been reported to vary from 3 to 12%; it has been recorded in 2.5% of spontaneous abortuses. The variation in reported frequency is affected by the variable size of the sample and the technique used for cord examination. Histologic sectioning is the most accurate way to identify a single umbilical artery.

The fetal anomalies associated with a single umbilical artery are variable, and often multiple, but they are not of any specific system or pattern except when a single umbilical artery is a part of a syndrome such as sironomelia. The single umbilical artery may be due to primary aplasia or to secondary atrophy.

Abnormalities of Insertion

Eccentric and Marginal Insertion

The normal patterns of cord insertion are eccentric insertion and central insertion. Eccentric insertion has been reported in over 50% of placentas and appears to have no clinical significance (Uyanwah-Akpom and Fox, 1977).

Marginal insertion is less common. Its reported incidence is from 2 to 15%. It is more common in spontaneous abortuses (Hathout, 1964) and in malformed fetuses, as well as in the intrauterine death of one of twins.

Fig. X-1. A thin, long cord with eccentric insertion in retained conception.

Fig. X-2. A short cord (2 cm) in a gestation with the limb body wall complex. Cord marked by arrows, L limbs, B bowel, T thorax, H head.

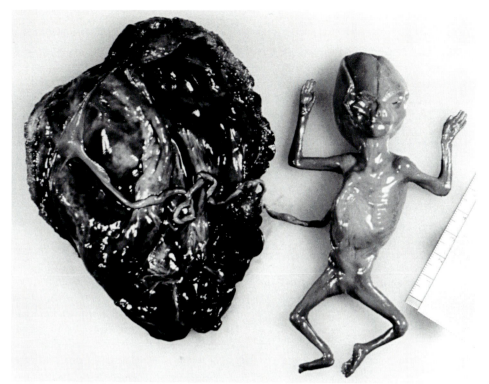

X-1

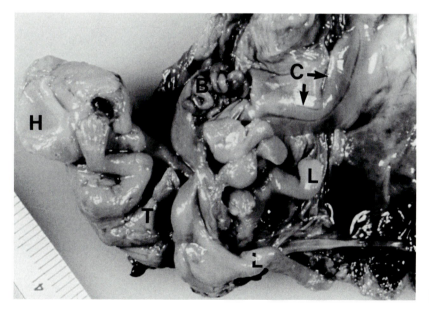

X-2

Velamentous Insertion

In this condition, the cord is inserted not into the placental disc but rather into the membranes. The incidence vary from less than 0.1 to 1.7% in multiple pregnancies (McLennan, 1968). An association between a velamentous insertion and a single umbilical artery has been noted. There is no evidence of increased spontaneous abortion (Philippe et al., 1968).

Mechanical Lesions of the Cord

Lesions include knots, rupture, torsion, and strictures. All are extremely rare in spontaneously aborted fetuses, although they are routinely described in texts on the pathology of the umbilical cord at birth (Fox, 1978; Benirschke and Driscoll, 1967).

Vascular Lesions

Edema

Edema of the cord is a common finding in spontaneously aborted, fresh or retained conceptuses. It is most commonly associated with fetal hydrops. The cord has a bloated swollen appearance throughout. On sectioning, edematous cord Wharton's jelly may seem to contain cystic spaces. Histologically, however, these are simply collections of fluid, without epithelial lining, in the ground substance of the cord. In retained pregnancies, the swelling of the cord may be focal rather than general.

Hematomas

Cord hematomas are a rare finding in a gestation under 20 weeks, except for traumatic lesions produced accidentally by a needle during amniocentesis or cordocentesis, and even these are infrequent. The hematomas are usually single and consist of an extravasation of blood into the Wharton's jelly. Although they can vary in size, cord hematomas prior to 20 weeks of gestation are usually small compared to those of term gestations, which may be quite large. Hematomas can be caused by the rupture of either an umbilical artery or vein.

Thrombosis of Umbilical Vessels

Thrombosis of cord vessels is usually described as a complication of cord compression, torsion, stricture, or hematoma in third-trimester pregnancies. It has not been observed in spontaneous abortions except as an iatrogenic complication of prenatal diagnosis (see hematomas).

Cysts

Two types of umbilical cord cysts can be observed in the previable fetus. One type represents a cystic enlargement of vestigial remnants (see above), the other consists of amniotic inclusions lined by an amniotic-type epithelium. Neither are considered clinically significant.

Fig. X-3. Edematous cord (arrow) in embryo (a) and large umbilical cord cysts (arrows) lined by amnion in macerated embryonic specimen (UL upper limb, LL lower limb) (b).

Fig. X-4. Edematous cord (arrow) in fetus.

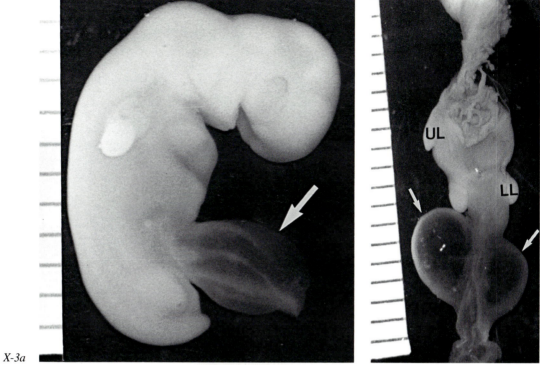

X-3a   *X-3b*

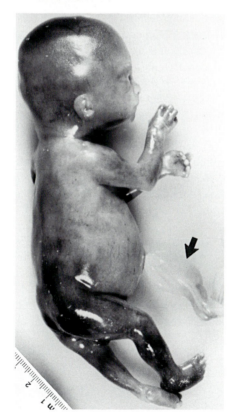

X-4

Placenta

Placental Size

For term placentas, the normal ratio of placental and fetal (P/F) weight has been established as 1/7. Placentas that are over 750 g or have a ratio of less than 1/7 are considered large; placentas with a ratio of more than 1/7 are considered small. As fetal weight varies during the previable period and many fetuses and placentas are retained for weeks prior to delivery following fetal death, severe fetal maceration and placental changes leading to reliable ratios for normal, large, or small placentas are not available. Approximate placental weights for each developmental week are given in Appendix T, Table II-6. Ultrasonography data on the relationship between placental and fetal growth are available (Wolfe et al., 1989).

Developmental Abnormalities

The most common developmental abnormalities of the placenta consist of variations of shape from the normal discoid form and, except for placenta membranacea, are simply variants with no apparent clinical significance. They are not associated with an increase of spontaneous abortions. *Bilobed* or *multilobed placentas* occur in 0.25 to 1.5% of pregnancies (Shanklin, 1978). The smaller lobe of the bilobed placenta is larger than one half the size of the larger lobe. *Accessory lobes* are areas of noninvolution of the chorion laeve, supplied by blood vessels from the main body of the placenta. They occur in about 7% of placentas.

Placenta membranacea is a gestational sac in which the villus tissue has not involuted in the area of chorion laeve. Thus, the greater area that is covered with villous tissue impairs sac expansion. Premature separation of the placenta resulting in fetal loss is a common complication. Fortunately, this anomaly is rare.

In *extrachorial placentation*, the chorionic plate from which the villi arise is smaller than the basal plate, and the transition from villous to nonvillous chorion takes place not at the placental margin but rather some distance within the circumference of the fetal surface of the placenta. *Circummarginate placenta*, a more common type of extrachorial placenta, has membranes coming off from inside the chorionic disc rather than the periphery. This is observed in 5 to 20% of placentas and is not thought to predispose to spontaneous abortion. *Circumvallate placenta* resembles the circummarginate variant but has a fold of membranes at the edge where the membranes come off from inside the chorionic disc; it represents a less common type of extrachorial placenta. Only 0.5 to 2% of term placentas have this morphology. Again, this variation in placental shape has not been associated with increased fetal loss, although it is associated with reduced numbers of fetal chorionic surface vessels and, thus, is likely to be a more serious anomaly during the later gestation.

Vascular Lesions

Because the placenta is nourished by maternal blood, problems with maternal blood flow have a significant effect on placental function and fetal growth and viability.

Premature Separation of the Placenta

Premature separation of part or all of the implanted placenta may occur prior to 20 weeks of gestation, but it is not as common as closer to term (one in 50 to 300 deliveries). Small zones of premature separation of the gestational sac, especially over the membranes or around the margin of the disc, are more common than large lesions and are of minimal clinical significance. Large zones of premature separation of the disc are a more serious threat to the continuation of the pregnancy; they are often called *abruptio placentae*. Prematurely separated placentas associated with spontaneous abortion usually have large blood clots attached to the maternal surface, with hemorrhage into the subchorionic space. The age of the clots can be estimated microscopically. In a fresh hemorrhage, red blood cells predominate, but after 36 hours, more and more fibrin appears. By 48 hours, neutrophils have appeared at the margin of the hematoma, and, from 5 to 7 days, pigment-laden macrophages infiltrate the basal plate of the placental floor villi and maternal decidua. Decidua overlying the hamatoma is often necrotic.

Fig. X-5. (a) Abruptio placentae with retroplacental hemorrhage, fetal surface (arrow). (b) Retroplacental hemorrhage, maternal surface (arrow).

Fig. X-6. Placental infarct with a marginal subchorionic hemorrhage (arrow).

Fig. X-7. Placental retention.

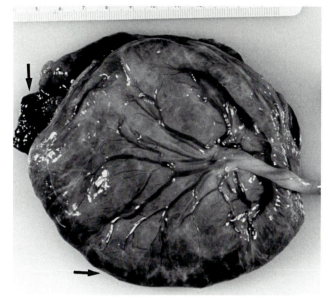

X-5a

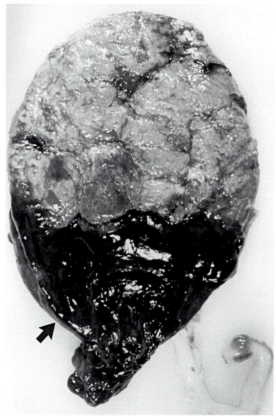

X-5b

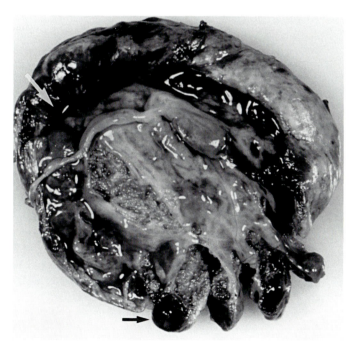

X-6

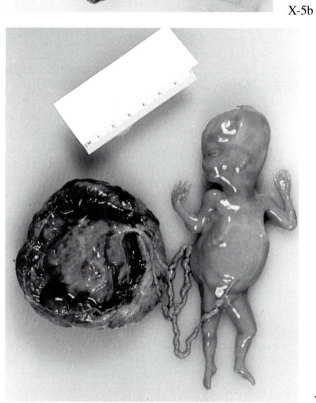

X-7

Infarcts

An infarct is a wedge-shaped lesion, usually with its apex directed toward the placental fetal surface and its base in continuity with the placental floor. Fresh infarcts are red; later, they become yellow and then white. Infarcts are more common at the margin of the placenta. Their significance depends on their number, size, time of occurrence, and the level of maternal blood flow. Part of the problem in assessing the significance of infarcts as a cause of fetal death is that maternal blood flow decreases after fetal death and some infarcts may have occurred after fetal death, rather than before.

Impaired maternal blood flow (also called *uteroplacental ischemia*) and retroplacental hemorrhage are related to placental infarcts. Affected placentas show either a minimum of 5% villous infarction or an old laminated hemorrhage on the maternal surface. In such placentas, Rushton (1988) has also described lesions in the placental bed, which consist of fibrinoid necrosis and an acute atherosis of the spiral arteries. Uteroplacental ischemia and retroplacental hemorrhage are detected in both macerated fetuses (16%) and fresh fetuses (20%).

Maternal Floor Infarction

This lesion, first described by Benirschke and Driscoll (1967), is the result of cessation of circulation through the villous vessels. In spontaneous abortion, the extent of the lesion is related to the duration of retention of the conceptus after embryonic or fetal death. The characteristic features of maternal floor infarction are a perivillous deposition of fibrin in the basal plate, which extends toward the chorionic plate to obliterate the intervillous space as the fibrin envelops the villi, and the villi, which are fibrotic, with vascular obliteration throughout the placenta.

Placental Changes Following Intrauterine Fetal Death

The fetal circulation ceases following fetal death in utero. This does not affect placental cells survival, since the maternal circulation within the intervillous space is maintained. However, the maternal–placental exchange decreases, and there are larger areas of perivillous fibrinosis. Perivillous fibrin depositions are most marked close to the placental floor, hence the term *maternal floor infarction*. Subchorionic hemorrhages, called *Breus moles*, are usually extensive and

recent; they show no evidence of organization. On gross examination, the retained placenta is firm and pale. The main histologic features are capillary collapse, stromal fibrosis, and sclerosis of the fetal stem arteries. There is an increase in villous syncytial knots, a thickening of the trophoblast basement membrane, and focal calcifications. Unfortunately, these changes may mask an underlying lesion that may have contributed to the death of the fetus.

Trophoblastic Disease

Although trophoblastic disease encompasses complete and partial hydatidiform moles and choriocarcinoma, only hydatidiform moles will be described.

The complete hydatidiform mole is characterized by a large "bunch of grapes" placenta without a detectable embryo or fetus. Microscopically, it is distinguished by trophoblastic hyperplasia, villous edema and the absence of any embryonic red blood cells (Szulman, 1988). The complete mole originates at fertilization in an androgenetic diploidy (46 chromosomes of paternal origin only). It is believed that this paternal chromosomal complement cannot support the development of the embryo beyond 2 to 3 weeks. Therefore, no embryo is ever found in the usually massive specimen of a complete hydatidiform mole.

The partial hydatidiform mole is characterized by a cystic placenta, which presents focal trophoblastic hyperplasia and focal villous swelling, and an embryo or a fetus. The partial mole has a triploid karyotype, with an extra haploid set of paternal origin. The diagnosis of the partial mole is more difficult than that of the complete mole, since the focal microscopic swelling of the villi varies in degree. The embryo and fetus in the partial mole present typical features (Chapters VIII and IX) of chromosomal triploidy.

Miscellaneous Lesions of the Placenta

Cyst(s) may be seen throughout the placenta. On the chorionic surface, they may be amniotic cysts or trophoblastic cysts. In the villous tissue, there may be cystic dilation of the stem villi, as seen in triploidy, or trophoblastic cysts in stem villi. Maternal lakes may grossly appear as cysts, but they are not true cysts, nor is the central liquefaction of an intervillous thrombus a cyst. Rarely, the residual gestational sac of an involuted conceptus of a multiple gestation may be present as a "cyst" on the chorionic surface.

Calcifications are usually a few millimeters in size, yellow-white, and firm; they are predominantly basal or scattered and are most frequently seen in retained products of conception. They are thought to be of no consequence.

Multiple Pregnancies

The multiple gestation rate is between one in 40 and one in 120. It is more common in Blacks and less common in Orientals, as compared to Caucasians.

Monozygotic twins originating from a single fertilized ovum occurs in 25% of twins. The frequency of monozygotic twinning is constant throughout the world. Dizygotic twinning refers to the fertilization of two separate ova; its frequency is affected by genetic factors.

A detailed examination of the placenta allows a categorization of multiple pregnancies, and its principles are described in standard texts; see, for example, *The Pathology of the Human Placenta*, by Benirschke and Driscoll (1967).

Fetus Papyraceus

A fetus papyraceus is a compressed, flattened, involuted twin fetus in pregnancies in which the other twin is developing normally. It has been described in the presence of both monochorionic and fused dichorionic placentas. The presence of a dead twin can elevate both alphafetoprotein and acetylcholinesterase levels in the amniotic fluid and falsely indicate the presence of fetal malformations (Winsor et al., 1987).

Acardia

This sporadic malformation is confined to one of the fetuses in a monochorionic multiple gestation. Acardiac fetuses differ greatly in appearance and degree of organogenesis. Most of them have an axis and lower limbs, with an absent or a malformed head. Various internal organs may be found, but the heart is absent or poorly developed. Their circulation is through the usually normal co-twin, triplet, or quintuplet by a return of reversed flow through direct artery to artery, or vein to vein, anastomoses of the cord or chorionic surface vessels.

Twin-to-Twin Transfusion Syndrome

This syndrome is due to an imbalanced blood flow through vascular anastomoses between the circulations of monochorionic twin fetuses. Anastomoses may be between larger vessels on the fetal placental surface or within the placental parenchyma. The net transfusion from one fetus to the other may be acute or chronic. In the acute pattern, the donor twin is usually pale, whereas the recipient twin is plethoric. In the chronic transfusion syndrome, there is discordant growth of the twins in weight and length. The smaller donor is anemic and the larger recipient is polycythemic.

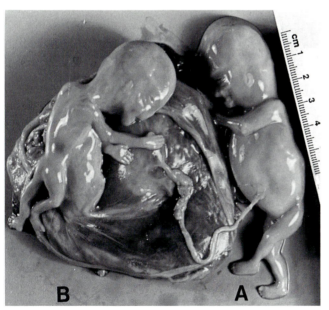
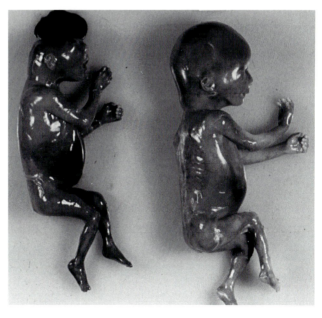

X-8   X-9

Fig. X-8. Macerated monozygous male twins with a normal twin A and a malformed twin B showing an absent umbilical cord and eventration of the abdominal viscera.

Fig. X-9. Male 16-week twins of undetermined zygosity with a normal karyotype and discrepancy for a neural tube closure defect.

Conjoined Twins

The incidence of monozygotic twin fusion is estimated to be one in 33,000 to one in 165,000 births; in 70% of these cases, fusion of the thorax (thoracopagus) is reported (Benirschke and Kim, 1973). The cause is not known, although incomplete fission of a single embryo affected by a variety of teratogens has been suggested. This condition is commonly diagnosed by ultrasound prior to 20 weeks of gestation and the pregnancy is usually terminated.

References

Altshuler G: The placenta, how to examine it, its normal growth and development, in *Perinatal Diseases*. Monograph of the International Academy of Pathology. Baltimore, Williams & Wilkins, 1981.

Benirschke K, Driscoll SF: *The Pathology of the Human Placenta*. Berlin, Heidelberg, New York, Springer-Verlag, 1967.

Benirschke K, Kim CK: Multiple pregnancy. *N Engl J Med* 288: 1329–1336, 1973.

Boyd JD, Hamilton WJ: *The Human Placenta*. Cambridge, W. Heffer, 1970.

Fox H: *Pathology of the Placenta*. London, Philadelphia, Toronto, Saunders, 1978.

Grange KD, Arya S, Opitz JM, Laxova R, Herrmann J, Gilbert EF: The short umbilical cord. *Birth Defects* OAS 23, 191–214, 1987.

Hathout H: The vascular pattern and mode of insertion of the umbilical cord in abortion material. *J Obstet Gynaecol Br Commonwealth* 71:963–964, 1964.

Johnson A, Uaper RJ, Barr MA, Corrido IL, Sherwood M, Coutinho W, Jackson L: Mosaicism in chorionic villous sampling: A predictor of poor perinatal outcome. *Obstetr Gynecol* In press.

Kalousek DK, Barrett IJ, McGillivray BC: Placental mosaicism and intrauterine survival of trisomies 13 and 15. *Am J Hum Genet* 44:338–343, 1989.

McLennan JE: Implications of the eccentricity of the human umbilical cord. *Am J Obstet Gynecol* 101:1124–1130, 1968.

Perrin EVD, Sander CH: How to examine the placenta and why, in *Pathology of the Placenta—Contemporary Issues in Surgical Pathology*. New York, Churchill-Livingstone, 1984.

Philippe E, Ritter J, Dehalleux JM, Renaud R, Gandar R: De la Pathologie des avortements spontanes. *Gynecol Obstet* 67:97–118, 1969.

Rushton DI: Placental pathology in spontaneous miscarriage in early embryonic death, in Beard RW and Sharp F (eds): *Early Pregnancy Loss: Mechanisms and Treatment*. Berlin Heidelberg New York, Springer-Verlag, 1988, pp 149–158.

Shanklin D: Anatomy of the placenta, in Falkner F, Tanner JM (eds): *Human Growth*. New York, Plenum Press, 1978, pp 333–353.

Szulman AE: The biology of trophoblastic disease: Complete and partial hydatidiform moles, in Beard RW and Sharp F (eds): *Early Pregnancy Loss*. Berlin Heidelberg New York, Springer-Verlag, 1988, pp 309–316.

Uyanwah-Akpom PO, Fox H: The clinical significance of marginal or velamentous insertion of the umbilical cord. *Br J Obstetr Gynaecol* 84:941–943, 1977.

Van Allen MI, Curry C, Callagher L: Limb body wall complex: I. Pathogenesis. *Am J Med Genet* 28:529–548, 1987.

Winsor EJT, St. John Brown B, Luther ER, Heifetz SA, Welch JP: Deceased co-twin as a cause of false positive fluid AFP and AChE. *Prenat Diagn* 7:485–489, 1987.

Wolf H, Oosting H, Treffers PE: A longitudinal study of the relationship between placental and fetal growth as measured by ultrasonography. *Am J Obstet Gynecol* 161:1140–1145, 1989.

Fig. X-10. A spontaneous abortion of twin pregnancy with one normal 12-week male fetus and one acardiac twin. The acardiac twin shows multiple developmental defects, including microcephaly, hypoplasia of the orbits and eyes and ears, absent nares, and a cleft lip. The extremities show some missing fingers and toes. There is a nuchal cystic hygroma, and numerous internal organs are missing. A cardiac organ was identified, but it contained a single chamber and had a single great vessel.

Fig. X-11. Omphalopagus-conjoined, 12-week female twins share a liver, the gut, and the umbilical cord. The twin labeled 46 shows complete situs inversus and a hypoplastic right heart.

Fig. X-12. A spontaneous abortion of a triplet pregnancy. All three fetuses are 15.5 weeks of development. The cause of the abortion could not be determined.

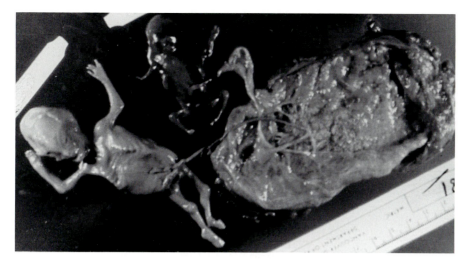

X-10

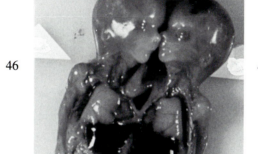

46   45

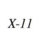

X-11

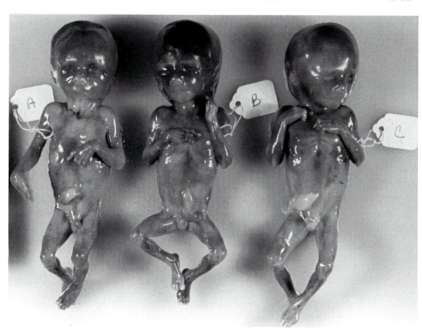

X-12

213

APPENDIX I

Confirmation of Prenatal Diagnosis

Confirmation of Prenatal Diagnosis

Prenatal diagnosis can be made by a noninvasive technique using ultrasound or by such invasive techniques as chorionic villus sampling, amniocentesis, fetoscopy, or fetal blood sampling. Fetal cells obtained by these methods are then used for cytogenetic, biochemical, and DNA studies.

Prenatal *ultrasound examination* was introduced in the 1950s. Most pregnancies in Western European countries and North America are now monitored by ultrasound when prenatal care is given. The benefits in terms of accurate assessment of gestational age, verification of fetal viability, detection of multiple pregnancies, placental localization, diagnosis of intrauterine growth retardation, and fetal abnormalities are well known. An accurate prenatal diagnosis of fetal abnormalities allows parents to make reproductive decisions on a more informed basis. A part of proper patient care is a detailed pathologic examination of the abnormal fetus in cases of pregnancy termination.

A study by Shen-Schwarz et al. (1989) showed that in 46% of 1961 cases of antenatal defect detection by ultrasound, important additional information was provided by the examination of the fetus from terminated pregnancies. In some cases, additional abnormalities were found at autopsy, which allowed syndrome diagnosis and correct genetic counseling. Oligohydroamnios and the death of the fetus in utero makes the ultrasound examination difficult, and autopsy in these cases is particularly important. In other cases, for example, a short-limbed dwarf, the study of the facial appearance and the bones make a precise diagnosis possible.

Chorionic villous sampling is a biopsy of 10–15 mg of chorion frondosum under ultrasound guidance usually at 9 to 11 weeks of gestation. The villi are cleared from decidua and utilized for cytogenetic analysis or for biochemical and DNA studies.

Amniocentesis for genetic indications evolved in the mid-1950s. It is performed around the 15th to the 16th week of gestation. At this time, the uterus is easily accessible by an abdominal approach and contains 200 to 250 ml of amniotic fluid. Under continuous ultrasound guidance, the needle is inserted into the amniotic sac and 20 ml of amniotic fluid, with both viable and nonviable cells, is withdrawn. Cells are utilized for further analysis after culturing.

Fetoscopy, an endoscopic intrauterine visualization of the fetus, has been used for prenatal diagnosis since 1973. It can also be used for *fetal blood sampling* in the second and third trimester. More recently, percutaneous ultrasound-guided needling of the placenta, umbilical cord, or fetal heart has been utilized. In this procedure the risks to the fetus are relatively small, and in highly specialized centers, the risks are only marginally greater than those of amniocentesis (Rodeck and Nicolaides, 1983).

For cytogenetic analysis, fetal cells from fetal blood, amniotic fluid, or chorionic villi can be cultured or a direct chromosomal preparation can be obtained from the cytotrophoblast. In all cases of pregnancy termination for prenatally detected chromosomal defects, a detailed fetal examination should be performed. Occasionally, the expected phenotype does not correspond to the cytogenetic prenatal diagnosis, in which case it is important to look for technical error and to repeat the karyotype analysis on both the fetus and the placenta to rule out mosaicism. To confirm prenatally detected mosaicism on either cultured amniotic fluid or chorionic villi, it is important to sample both the placenta and the fetus itself extensively. The placenta should be represented by a sample of villi, chorion, and amnion. The fetus, depending on its condition after delivery, can be sampled from skin and multiple internal organs if it is well preserved. An autolyzed fetus can best be sampled from any tendon, periosteum, or cartilage (Table 1).

When a diagnosis of the developmental defect has been made by biochemical (Table 2) or DNA analysis (Table 3), the pathologist must be ready to confirm the specific diagnosis, using fetal and placental tissues.

TABLE I.I-1. Specimen collection for prenatal diagnosis confirmation: Cytogenetics.

Fetus and placenta[a]	Samples for tissue culture
Typical phenotype for a diagnosed defect, e.g., trisomy 13	No samples needed; morphologic findings confirm prenatal diagnosis
No phenotype typical for diagnosed defect	Sample both fetus (skin or tendon or internal organ) and placenta (amnion or chorion or villi)
Prenatal diagnosis of mosaicism on chorionic villi, and amniocentesis	Sample extensively both fetus (blood, skin, tendon, and internal organs) and placenta (amnion, chorion, and villi)
Prenatal diagnosis of mosaicism in fetal blood	Sample fetal blood, if possible, and fetal skin, tendon, and internal organs

[a]If the fetus is severely macerated, use, for confirmatory studies, the placental tissue, including villi, amnion, and chorion.

TABLE I.I-2. Specimen collection for prenatal diagnosis confirmation: Biochemical studies.

1. The pathologist must know the specific disorder diagnosed prenatally that requires confirmation. Then the pathologist should contact the laboratory that made the original diagnosis and make arrangements to obtain the most suitable sample.
2. In general, viable fetal cells for fibroblast tissue culture are required.
3. In the case of defects of some urea cycle enzyme defects and glycogen storage diseases, a sample of liver tissue is needed, since these enzymes are not expressed in fibroblasts.
4. In chondrodysplasias, cultured and frozen cartilage may be needed to distinguish different subtypes.
5. Sampling for electron microscopy should be remembered, and specific tissues selected, depending on the specific disorders.

TABLE I.I-3. Specimen collection for prenatal diagnosis confirmation: Molecular studies.

1. The pathologist must know the specific disorder diagnosed prenatally, which requires confirmation.
2. In general, any fresh or frozen ($-20°C$ short-term, $-70°C$ long-term) embryonic or fetal tissue is suitable for DNA extraction.
3. Cultured fibroblasts from any embryonic or fetal tissue are an excellent source of DNA.
4. For some disorders diagnosed by DNA, such as β-thalassemia, a morphologic diagnosis of fetal hydrops, liver enlargement and hemoglobin electrophoresis are sufficient confirmation.

SELECTION AND HANDLING OF MATERIAL FOR CHROMOSOME ANALYSIS

1. The specimens are handled aseptically using sterile forceps, scissors, and disposable sterile Petri dishes.
2. If the conceptus is less than 8 weeks developmental age, the amnion, chorion, and chorionic villi with decidua removed are the most suitable tissues for the initiation of tissue culture.
3. If the previable fetus is fresh, fetal heart blood is suitable for lymphocyte culture. This should be backed up by a piece of fetal skin or amnion.
4. Amnion, chorion, or villi are the most suitable specimens if the fetus is degenerated. If the placenta is not available, tendon, muscle, cartilage, or periosteum can be used.
5. Except for fetal blood, all specimens are washed in three separate Petri dishes containing 1% Antibiotic-Antimycotic in normal saline. The tissues are then placed in minimal essential media ready for transporting to the Cytogenetic Laboratory.

References

Shen-Schwartz S, Neish C, Hill L: Antenatal ultrasound for fetal anomalies. *Pedr Pathol* 9:1–9, 1989.

Rodeck CH, Nicolaides KH: Ultrasound guided invasive procedures in obstetrics. *Clin Obstetr Gynaecol* 10:515–520, 1983.

Nicolaides KH, Campbell S: Diagnosis of fetal abnormalities by ultrasound, in Milunsky A (ed): *Genetic Disorders and the Fetus*, ed 2. New York, London, Plenum Press, 1986, pp 521–570.

Color Plates

Fig. I-6. A well-preserved, triploid, Stage 18 embryo is attached to the chorionic sac. A large parietal encephalocele (arrow) and an open neural tube defect in caudal region (arrow) can be seen.

Fig. I-7. A damaged, trisomy 14 embryo, with significantly delayed development of the upper and lower limb. Microcephaly, eye coloboma, and midface dysplasia are also present.

Fig. I-8. A degenerated abnormal embryo, Stage 23, with wide-open eyes, a bilateral cleft lip, and a bilateral postaxial polydactyly (arrows).

Fig. I-9. A normal 14-week fetus in an intact amniotic sac with amniotic fluid. The ruptured chorionic membrane is indicated by arrows.

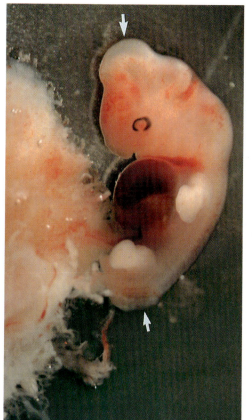

I-6

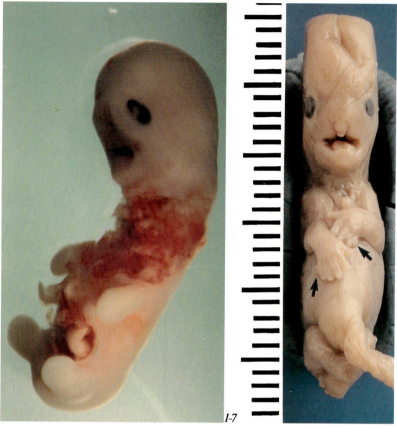

I-7   *I-8*

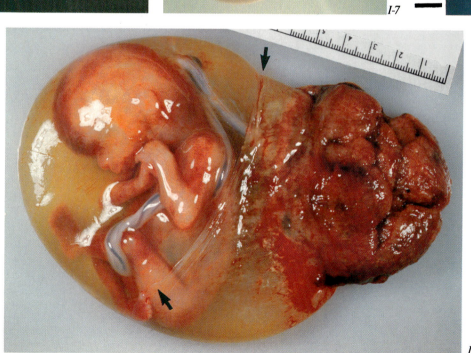

I-9

Fig. I-10. A well-preserved, 16-week female fetus, with trisomy 18. The craniofacial and skeletal malformed anomalies include a small mandible, an abnormal external ear, a hypoplastic and abnormally positioned left thumb, a right club hand with an absent thumb and hypoplasia of the radius and ulna, and rocker-bottom feet. In addition, there is a large omphalocele that contains most of the abdominal organs.

Fig. I-11. A well-preserved, 14- to 15-week male fetus, with a multiple lethal pterygium syndrome. Note the cystic hygroma, clubfeet, and pterygia (axillary, antecubital, popliteal, and chin-chest) (arrows).

Fig. I-12. A 16-week fetus with acrania. Note the complete absence of the scalp and skull bones.

Fig. I-13. A degenerated, formaldehyde-fixed, 9½-week fetus, with bilateral absence of radia and thumbs. There is also a bifid toe on the left foot (arrow).

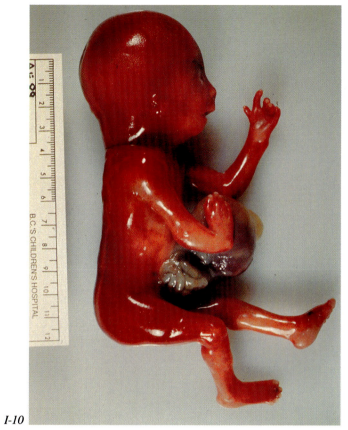

I-10

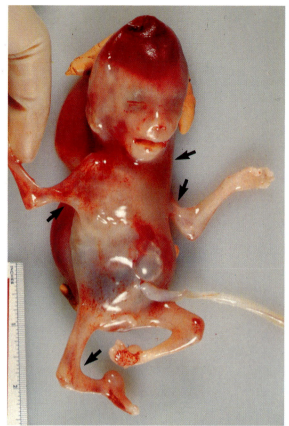

I-11

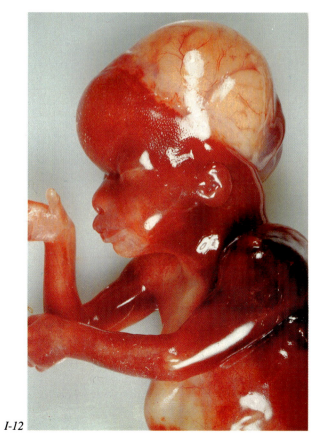

I-12

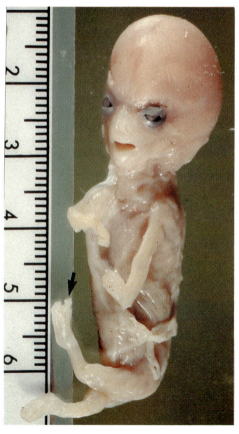

I-13

Fig. I-14. An Alizarin Red S preparation of a fetal forearm and hand, showing an absent radius and thumb.

Fig. I-15. Bilateral dysplastic cystic kidneys in an 18-week female fetus; A, adrenals; arrows, cystic kidneys.

Fig. I-16. A severely macerated, 13-week female fetus with an extensive retroperitoneal tumor (arrows) consisting of fragmented brain tissue. No developmental anomalies were identified; the karyotype was 46,XX.

Fig. I-17. A degenerated, 10½-week male fetus, with the amnion-rupture sequence. There is an irregular bizarre facial clefting and digital amputations and constrictions (arrows). In addition, there is a large omphalocele (O).

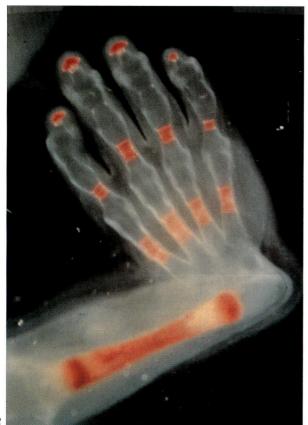

I-14

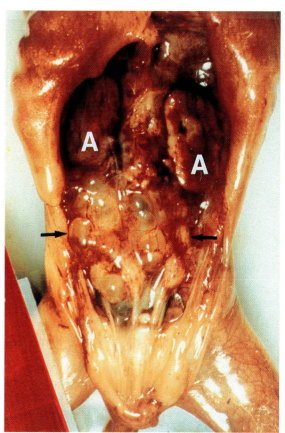

I-15

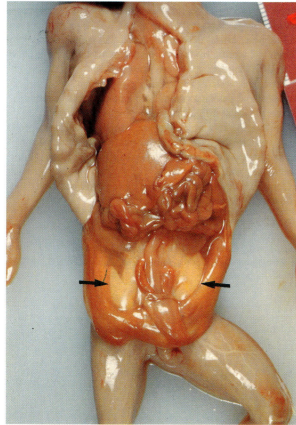

I-16

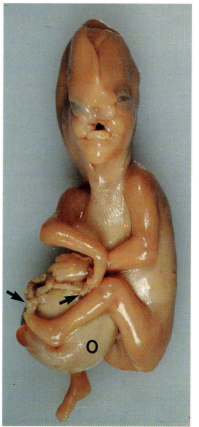

I-17

TABLE II.3. Hand and Foot Lengths Correlated with Developmental Age in Previable Fetuses.

Developmental age (weeks)	Hand length (mm)	Foot length (mm)
11	10	12
	±2	±2
12	15	17
	±2	±3
13	18	19
	±1	±1
14	19	22
	±1	±2
15	20	25
	±3	±3
16	26	28
	±2	±2
17	27	29
	±3	±4
18	29	33
	±2	±2

Modified from McBride ML, Baillie J, Poland BJ. Growth parameters in normal fetuses. *Teratology* 29:185–201, 1984; supplemented with previously unpublished data.

TABLE II.4. Relation between Developmental State and Palatal Closure[a] in 225 Human Embryos and Early Fetuses.

CRL (mm)	Total cases (no.)	Number Closed	Number Open	Percent with palate closed
24.0–25.9	9	0	9	0
26.0–27.9	13	0	13	0
28.0–29.9	10	1	9	10.0
30.0–31.9	12	1	11	8.3
32.0–33.9	11	1	10	9.1
34.0–35.9	10	1	9	10.0
36.0–37.9	13	3	10	23.1
38.0–39.9	11	3	8	27.3
40.0–41.9	17	10	7	58.8
42.0–43.9	14	11	3	78.6
44.0–45.9	13	12	1	92.3
46.0–47.9	11	11	0	100.0
48.0–49.9	13	13	0	100.0
50.0–51.9	16	16	0	100.0
52.0–53.9	17	17	0	100.0
54.0–55.9	18	18	0	100.0
56.0–57.9	17	17	0	100.0

[a]Hand and soft palate completely closed (the uvula is not included) (stage of the closure of the human palate, by Tadchiko Iuzuka, personal communication to Dr. B. Poland)

TABLE II.5. Umbilical Cord Lengths for Normal Fetuses Developmental Ages 8 to 18 Weeks

Fetal age (weeks)	Number	Cord length (cm)	95% Confidence interval (cm)
8	3	6.4	5.2 – 7.7
9	6	8.0	7.0 – 9.1
10	7	9.7	8.7 – 10.6
11	8	11.3	10.5 – 12.1
12	15	12.9	12.2 – 13.6
13	12	14.5	13.9 – 15.1
14	12	16.1	15.5 – 16.7
15	8	17.7	17.1 – 18.4
16	9	19.4	18.6 – 20.1
17	9	21.0	20.5 – 21.4
18	3	22.6	21.5 – 23.7

Data from the Embryofetopathology Laboratory, B.C. Children's Hospital.

TABLE II.6. Placental Weights for Normal Fetuses, Developmental Ages 8 to 18 Weeks.

Fetal age (weeks)	Number	Placental weight (g)	95% Confidence interval (g)
8	2	1.6	0.0 – 3.7
9	7	15.2	13.3 – 17.0
10	10	28.8	27.2 – 30.4
11	9	42.4	41.1 – 43.8
12	14	56.1	54.8 – 57.3
13	17	69.7	68.4 – 71.0
14	15	83.3	81.8 – 84.8
15	12	96.9	95.2 – 98.6
16	11	110.5	108.5 – 112.5
17	14	124.2	121.8 – 126.5
18	4	137.8	135.0 – 140.5

Data from the Embryofetopathology Laboratory, B.C. Children's Hospital.

TABLE II.7.

EMBRYOFETOPATHOLOGY CONSULTATION REQUEST FORM	PATIENT INFORMATION

CLINICAL INFORMATION

MOTHER'S BIRTHDATE (IMPORTANT)

DR.

FROM HOSPITAL

1. PREVIOUS SPECIMENS: _____

LABORATORY	DATE	ACCESSIONS NUMBER

2. OBSTETRIC HISTORY: _____

GRAVIDA	PARA	ABORTION (THERAPEUTIC)	ABORTION (SPONTANEOUS)	STILLBIRTH

DETAILS FROM PREVIOUS ABORTIONS _____

_____

_____

3. CURRENT PREGNANCY: _____

D.L.N.M.P.	GESTATIONAL AGE

– bleeding _____

– illness _____

– drugs _____

– other _____

4. SPECIMEN ACQUISITION: _____

SPONTANEOUS	ELECTIVE/TECHNIQUE

DATE

5. OTHER SIGNIFICANT MEDICAL/SURGICAL HISTORY:

DATE REQUESTED	REQUESTING PHYSICIAN

TABLE II.8. Instructions for Mailing Aborted Tissue.

In order to ensure complete examination, morphologically, microbiologically and cytogenetically, the following instructions should be carried out:

1. The whole conceptus (everything aborted) should be submitted. This means the fetus and placenta and all the tissues spontaneously expelled or removed surgically by either a D & C or the suction method.

2. The aborted material should be placed in a clean container of appropriate size without additives.

3. Scant material should be kept moist by the naturally present blood or with a few milliliters of sterile normal saline.

4. Sterile technique should be used in preparing the specimen for transport.

5. The containers should be labeled appropriately and tightly sealed to prevent leakage.

6. Specimens shipped from long distance should be insulated with a cold pack. Do not freeze. To prevent tissue deterioration, the specimen should be sent immediately by postal service First Class, Special Delivery, or by Courier Service.

7. The requisition form should be completed and accompany the specimen. The clinical history is important for it is that information and the morphologic findings that dictate whether chromosome studies or other special tests are initiated.

TABLE II.9. Protocol for Fetal Examination.

1.

NAME: _____   CASE NO: _____

DOCTOR: _____   DATE: _____

HOSPITAL: _____

SOURCE: Therapeutic:

      Indication _____   Spontaneous:_____

      Method _____

ECTOPIC:

      Site _____

HISTORY: _____   Previous Specimen No. _____

      _____

      _____

SPECIAL PROCEDURES:

                          Date Performed _____

                          Result _____

      Photographs _____

      X-ray _____

      Cytogenetics
         Material Submitted _____

      Research tissue _____

      Dermatoglyphics _____

      Metabolic _____

      Microbiology
         Material Submitted:

         Viral _____

         Bacteria _____

      Electron microscopy _____

      Other _____

continued

TABLE II.9. *Continued.*

2.

CASE NO: _____

EXTERNAL EXAMINATION

FETUS: Intact   _____   Damaged   _____   Incomplete   _____

PLACENTA: Intact   _____   Ruptured   _____   Damaged   _____   Not
Received   _____

                    Incomplete   _____

CONDITION: Fresh   _____   GENERAL FEATURES: Edema   _____

                    Fixed   _____   Bruising   _____

                    Macerated _____   Petechiae   _____

                    Autolysed   Colour   _____

                    Degenerate   Other   _____

                    Weight _____ gms   SEX: Female _____   Male _____   Ambiguous _____

                    C.R.L. _____ cm   Gestation age _____

                    C.H.L. _____ cm   Developmental age _____

                    H.C. _____ cm   Method of assessment _____

                    Chest _____ cm   Other _____

HEAD AND NECK:

                    Shape   _____   Eyes   _____   Palate   _____

                    Neck   _____   Ears   _____   Tongue _____

                    Scalp   _____   Nose   _____   Mandible_____

                    Facies _____   Lips   _____   Other   _____

VERTEBRAL COLUMN: _____

TRUNK: Anterior _____   Perineum_____

                    Posterior _____   Genitalia _____   Anus   _____

EXTREMITIES: Shoulders   _____   Pelvis   _____

                              Arms   _____   Legs   _____

                              Hands   _____   Feet   _____

                              Fingers   _____   Toes   _____

continued

Table II.9. *Continued.*

3.

CASE NO. _____

INTERNAL EXAMINATION

CONDITION:	Preservation _____	Organ Orientation _____
	Intact _____	Diaphragm _____
	Damaged _____	Other _____
HEAD AND NECK:	Thyroid _____	Other _____
	Neck Structures _____	

RESPIRATORY TRACT: (R) Lung – Fissures _____   (L) Lung – Fissures _____

(R) Lung – Lobation _____   (L) Lung – Lobation _____

Tracheobronchial Tree _____   Pleura _____

Other _____
_____

GASTROINTESTINAL: Esophagus _____   Anus _____

Small bowel _____   Gallbladder _____

Rectum _____   Duodenum _____

Liver _____   Colon _____

Stomach _____   Mesenteries _____

Cecum _____   Pancreas _____

Other _____
_____

RETICULO-
ENDOTHELIAL: Thymus _____   Spleen _____

Bone marrow _____   Other _____

ADRENALS: _____
_____

continued

TABLE II.9. *Continued.*

4.

CASE NO. _____

INTERNAL EXAMINATION

CARDIOVASCULAR
SYSTEM: Systemic arteries _____   Pulmonaries _____

               Systemic veins _____   Pulmonary veins _____

               Coronaries _____   Configuration _____

               Aortic arch _____   Major branches _____

HEART: R.A.   _____   L.A.   _____   F.O.   _____

               T.V.   _____   M.V.   _____   Ductus arteriosus   _____

               R.V.   _____   L.V.   _____   Endocardium   _____

               Conus _____   I.V.S. _____   Myocardium   _____

               P.V.   _____   A.V.   _____   Pericardium   _____

               Atrial septum _____

               Other _____

continued

TABLE II.9. *Continued.*

5.

CASE NO. _____

URINARY TRACT: Kidneys (left) _____   Bladder _____   External _____

    (right) _____   Ureters _____

    Other _____

GENITALIA: Gonads _____   Internal _____   External _____

CENTRAL   Brain
NERVOUS SYSTEM: (not examined) _____   Spinal Cord _____

    Other _____   Pituitary (see report) _____

PLACENTA: Complete _____   Size _____

    Fragmented _____   Weight _____

CORD: Measurement _____   Description _____

    Insertion _____   Vessels _____

AMNIOTIC FLUID _____

MEMBRANES _____

FETAL SURFACE _____

MATERNAL SURFACE _____

PARENCHYMA _____

GROSS DIAGNOSIS _____

_____

_____

_____

_____

_____

_____

_____

_____

continued

TABLE II.9. *Continued.*

6.

CASE NO. _____

TISSUE SECTIONED	WEIGHT (g)	NORMAL WEIGHT (g)	HISTOLOGIC FINDINGS
_____ Thymus			
_____ Thyroid			
_____ Lungs			
_____ Heart			
_____ Liver			
_____ Spleen			
_____ Pancreas			
_____ Kidneys			
_____ Adrenals			
_____ Gonads			
_____ Brain			
_____ Bone			
_____ Other			
_____ Placenta			

SPECIAL STAINS:

BONE MEASUREMENTS: Humerus _____ mm   Forearm _____ mm   Hand _____ mm

Femur _____   Lower leg _____ mm   Foot _____ mm

Other _____

_____

_____

Index